The
Good News
About the Bad News

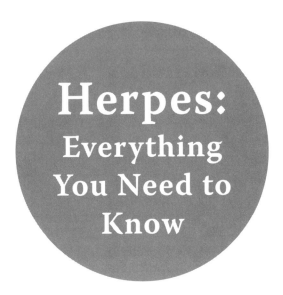

Herpes:
Everything
You Need to
Know

TERRI WARREN, RN, NP

New Harbinger Publications, Inc.

Publisher's Note

Distributed in Canada by Raincoast Books

Copyright © 2009 by Terri Warren
New Harbinger Publications, Inc.
5674 Shattuck Avenue
Oakland, CA 94609
www.newharbinger.com

FSC
Mixed Sources
Product group from well-managed
orests and other controlled sources

Cert no. SW-COC-002283
www.fsc.org
© 1996 Forest Stewardship Council

All Rights Reserved
Printed in the United States of America

Acquired by Melissa Kirk; Cover design by Amy Shoup
Edited by Nelda Street; Text design by Tracy Marie Carlson

Library of Congress Cataloging-in-Publication Data

Warren, Terri.
  The good news about the bad news : herpes, everything you need to know / Terri Warren.
    p. cm.
  Includes bibliographical references.
  ISBN-13: 978-1-57224-618-8 (pbk. : alk. paper)
  ISBN-10: 1-57224-618-9 (pbk. : alk. paper)
  1. Herpesvirus diseases--Popular works. I. Title.
  QR201.H48W37 2009
  616.9'112--dc22

                                2009007492

11 10 09   10 9 8 7 6 5 4 3 2 1   First printing

I dedicate this book to my dear friend Doug Hilton. Doug, you had better live to see this book published. Let's share something from Ponzi to celebrate.

Contents

Foreword

I'm pleased to have the opportunity to introduce this book. While I was reviewing the manuscript for scientific accuracy and medical completeness, I was struck by Terri's ability to accurately educate her readers about herpes infection while reassuring her audience they would have full and satisfying lives in spite of having herpes. I think this book will be very useful both to people who have herpes and to those who are concerned about herpes in partners or loved ones.

Terri has done an outstanding job of making the book readable for the layperson but thorough enough to be a valuable resource for professionals, whether they are medical clinicians or counselors. As a physician and herpes researcher, I find it difficult to put myself in the position of the layperson trying to understand this infection for the first time, but I'm confident that the book's down-to-earth style and well-defined concepts will make it a very accessible resource that readers will pick up again and again. Terri has taken concepts that will certainly be confusing to many people (like asymptomatic shedding of the herpes virus) and explained them in ways that nonmedical and medical people alike can understand. I hope providers who counsel clients with herpes will take note of her approach to these complex topics and use this style in their everyday practice.

Armed with the knowledge gained from this compassionate book, readers with herpes will be reassured that they can cope with their condition, and herpes will take its appropriate role as one of those issues in life that is challenging but can be managed successfully.

—Kenneth H. Fife, MD, Ph.D.
Professor of Medicine
Indiana University School of Medicine

Acknowledgments

I would like to thank the following people who have been with me as I wrote this book.

Hal, who good-naturedly read each chapter and gave valuable input as we flew around the United States day after day in a big silver tube, preaching the gospel of good herpes care to any clinician who would listen.

My daughters, for being patient when I sometimes didn't have time for them while I did this instead. Now I have time again.

Ken Fife, for reviewing each chapter so carefully for accuracy, and for giving feedback in such a hearable way.

Jim Catano, who helped me with editing throughout the writing of the book.

My literary agent, Lilly Ghahremani, who helped me through difficult times with her kindness and consistency.

Zane Brown, who has guided my thoughts on the care of women with herpes and their babies for twenty-five years now.

Betsy O'Rourke, my colleague at WebMD, for reviewing chapters and giving thoughtful input on patient-related issues.

Lisa Gilbert, for reviewing chapters with an eye toward patient advocacy.

My best friend, Jane Hilton, for helping me get through writing this book while her own life was turned upside down.

Larry Corey, Anna Wald, Peter Leone, Larry Stanberry, Paul Griffiths, Rich Whitely, Steve Straus, Charlie Ebel, Steve Sacks, and many others who taught me about herpes over the years—bless you for sharing your wisdom with me.

The patients in my clinic and the herpes support group, both online and in person, who have taught me so much about what's important to you, what you need, and how you can best be helped to live fully with herpes.

Introduction

Whew! Buying this book about herpes was a *big* step! Good for you! Some of you purchased it on the Internet, knowing it would be shipped to you without a hint as to the content. Others found it in a bookstore. If you bought it in person, maybe you were hesitant about asking the clerk for titles on this subject. Did you buy a few other books at the same time so that this one "blended in"? Was it like buying condoms or tampons at the grocery store—maybe you also buy potato chips and a celebrity-gossip magazine so that such personal items aren't as obvious?

Welcome to the much-misunderstood world of genital herpes! It's a subject most people don't feel comfortable with, no matter where they live or who they are. Thanks to recurring TV commercials, I think we now feel a bit more comfortable talking about things like erectile dysfunction and urinary frequency—and yes, even genital herpes. The number of people who have herpes surprises most everyone. There are more people with genital herpes than with erectile dysfunction and urinary frequency *combined*. There are even more people with genital herpes than with either diabetes or high blood pressure! About one in every five adults in the United States has genital herpes (Xu et al. 2006). Amazingly, almost 90 percent of the people who have it don't know they have it (Xu et al. 2006). So if you *know* you have herpes—and you or someone you care about probably does since you're reading a book about it—you're clearly the exception and not the rule.

Erectile dysfunction (ED), bladder problems, and herpes all involve that part of the body we tend to be nervous talking about—the mysterious area between waist and thigh. For most people, it's quite a challenge to talk about genital problems. And that publicly held neurosis makes herpes a more difficult issue than just the medical condition itself. When you were first diagnosed, you may have wondered what the future would bring and worried about how the people around you would react. We can't quickly change society's negative notions about this problem. Hopefully, however, I can change *your* attitudes and *your* level of knowledge about it. That's what this book is all about: to make you more informed about this virus, to help you feel more empowered about having herpes, to give you more control over passing the infection to sex partners, to describe treatment options, and most importantly, to help you learn to accept and respect yourself or other people who have herpes.

Since 1982, I've run a private sexually transmitted infection (STI) clinic in Portland, Oregon. As you might imagine, very little about people's sex lives and their genitalia surprises me anymore. This applies particularly to genital herpes. In addition to seeing thousands of STI patients every year, our clinic has run more than 120 research studies—most of them about oral or genital herpes—evaluating things like new treatments, new diagnostic tests, and new vaccines. Since 1999, I've also been the WebMD herpes resident expert, answering questions daily about herpes. (WebMD is the largest online source for medical information: www.WebMD.com.) These questions range from "How do I interpret these particular blood-test results?" to "Can my eight-year-old get herpes by digging through the laundry basket for his favorite T-shirt if my underwear is in there too?" Answering these questions every day keeps my finger on the pulse of the herpes world.

Last year I asked myself, "Where are these WebMD posters getting their information?" There was only a handful of books about herpes on the market. But compared to the number of publications on hypertension or diabetes, books on herpes were rare. That shortage of truly helpful books on the topic led me to write this one. I believe you need information that's easy to understand but complex enough to satisfy your need to know the details.

In the first chapter, I'll address the top ten questions people ask about genital herpes, offering a kind of late-night TV talk show summary about this infection, and I'll tell you where in the book you can find more details on these questions.

In chapter 2, we'll talk about the eight different herpes viruses that can infect humans. "Herpes" means genital herpes to most people, but the herpes simplex virus has seven siblings. I'll give you all the scuttle-butt about this family called "Herpes."

Chapter 3 addresses the difficult topic of transmission to a sexual partner. If herpes weren't infectious to other people through sex, there'd really be very little concern about it. But it is, so we'll talk about the risks, the odds, and the ways to reduce the chances of giving herpes to a partner. We'll also discuss how herpes impacts sexuality.

An accurate diagnosis of herpes is the foundation of everything that comes afterward. Yet, to use a football metaphor, this diagnosis gets "fumbled" more often than you'd think. Chapter 4 gives you a clear summary of the best diagnostic tools, their limitations, timing, uses, and cost, and we'll have a good discussion about the misdiagnosis of genital herpes.

Women have special concerns about herpes: the risk of passing it to a baby during pregnancy, delivery, or both is scary, and so are the nasty rumors about a link with cervical cancer. We'll discuss realities and dispel myths about these topics in chapter 5.

In chapter 6, we look at treatment options. Did you know that before 1982, there was no treatment available at all for herpes? Now there are three good drugs, with more on the way, and vaccines for both prevention and treatment are being studied. We'll also touch on alternative treatments in this chapter.

Are you nervous about the prospective of telling a future partner that you have genital herpes? Well, join the group and get information about how to handle that challenging task in chapter 7. I've got some really good tips for talking about herpes successfully.

In chapter 8, we'll discuss the emotional, psychological, and relationship concerns associated with genital herpes: the sick feeling in the pit of your stomach when you first hear the diagnosis, the bad jokes, and the emotions that may follow, such as guilt, shame, loss, isolation, and, finally, acceptance.

Chapter 9 will tackle the relationship between HIV and HSV 2. If both viruses exist in the same person, they make each other more troublesome; I'll tell you why and how.

Since herpes isn't the only STI around, in chapter 10 we'll review the other STIs commonly found in the United States.

And finally, in chapter 11, I share some resources for learning more about herpes so that you can stay current on the topic.

This isn't a science book; it's a people book. I'll give you clear and accurate facts, but I'll also address your feelings. This is a book that I hope you'll refer back to regularly over the years. You can give it to potential partners after you've had "the talk" so that they have accurate information on which to base the decision of whether to make sex a part of your relationship. And you can even give this little volume to family members if you decide to tell them you have herpes, so they'll know you're really going to be okay.

This is a casual and friendly book. Like most people, I learn things best when facts are presented in easy-to-understand terms with lots of examples. When I was in school, I used to wonder, "Why do they use the term 'erythema' when they mean 'red'? Why say 'edema' for 'swollen'? Why do we use 'fissure' when 'skin crack' will do?" For me, the simple terms are always best when learning about an unfamiliar subject. Technical medical words can even put distance between medical professionals and their patients. But in this book, I hope you feel as if we're sitting somewhere discussing this together. I hope this book is a personal experience for you and a resource you can use whenever you need reassurance, comfort, or just more information.

When you finish this book, you'll know more about herpes than you did before—or may have ever wanted to know! And you'll have the tools necessary to find more information if you need it. I'll be right there with you in spirit as you study these chapters. If I could sit next to you and answer your questions or hold your hand if you get sad or anxious, I would. But, short of that, I know that reading this book will help you live better with genital herpes.

Chapter 1

The Top Ten Questions About Genital Herpes: Everything You Always Wanted to Know but Were Afraid to Ask

One late-night talk-show host is famous for his top-ten lists. I hope he won't mind, but I'm going to borrow his idea. Here's my top-ten list of questions asked most often about genital herpes. They come from patients at my clinic and from the WebMD message board. And if your question isn't in here, I bet you'll find it farther along in the book.

1. How did I get genital herpes? Herpes is passed from one person to another through sexual contact. You get it from someone who has herpes through intercourse, receiving oral or anal sex, or genital to genital rubbing. You don't get it from touching doorknobs or sharing blue jeans or toilet seats—unless, of course, you're having sex on a toilet seat, but that's for a whole different book.

A closely related, often-asked question is, "Could I have gotten herpes through a sexual encounter that didn't involve intercourse?" Lap dancing, oral sex, genital rubbing, and mutual masturbation are all alive and well, and occur with great frequency. Sometimes these activities happen with people who aren't regular partners or spouses, and that can create concerns about the risk of getting an *STI* (*sexually transmitted infection*). First, let me assure you with complete certainty that you can't get genital herpes while you have your clothes on and someone is "dancing" on your lap. It doesn't even matter if there's moisture present. The virus doesn't somehow "wick" through fabric and infect the genitals. When the clothes come off, however, and genitals are rubbing directly together, there *is* a chance of getting herpes. And the real risk of getting genital herpes during a single sexual encounter is very low, but it's not zero. Receiving oral sex also presents some risk too, but now the risk changes to one of being infected with the cold-sore virus, *herpes simplex virus type 1 (HSV 1)*, in the genital area. HSV 1 (very often, oral herpes) can be transmitted from the mouth of one person to the genitals of a sex partner through oral sex, even if the giver doesn't have an active cold sore.

And finally, what about when one person masturbates another? This is truly safe sex as far as herpes is concerned. Unless someone has a herpes lesion on his or her hand, which is so rare it's not worth even considering, masturbation presents no risk for transmission. "Okay," you say, "but what if the person touches his or her genitals and then touches mine?" Again, the risk is so low; don't spend any time and energy even worrying about it. I'll talk a whole lot more about transmission and sexuality in chapter 3.

2. Now that I have herpes, can I ever have sex again?

Yes, you definitely can, but I'm not going to mislead you by saying that sex will be the same as it was before. There's a risk of giving herpes to an uninfected partner, and you need to deal head-on with that issue. First, you should tell all future partners about your herpes before you have sex so that they can make educated decisions about their risk of getting infected. It may be difficult to tell your partner, but you'll know in your heart that it's the right thing to do. If your partner doesn't have herpes (and he or she would need a blood test to know for sure), he or she will be vulnerable to getting herpes from you. Daily herpes medication and condoms greatly reduce the risk of transmission, but neither offers absolutely perfect prevention—not even when used together. If your partner already has the same type of herpes you do, then you *can* have sex just as you did before you had herpes. I'll tell you more about how to break the news to partners in chapter 7, and we'll talk about medicines for herpes in chapter 6.

3. Will genital herpes shorten my life? That one's easy—*absolutely not*! In years past, there was concern that herpes might be linked to cervical cancer, but we know now that *human papillomavirus (HPV)*, not herpes, causes cervical cancer. I know—it's easy to get all those viruses that begin with *H* mixed up. I'll talk more about women's special health concerns in chapter 5.

4. Can herpes be cured? Right now, there's no known cure for herpes. But in 1981 there wasn't even a treatment for herpes, so look how far we've come already! Now we have three very good medicines, so you just never know what might develop. There are two kinds of herpes vaccines being studied right now. One is designed to prevent herpes infection, and the other to treat herpes, so those are promising projects. Keep in mind, however, that there are many conditions with no known cure: diabetes, hypertension, HIV, and thyroid disease, to name just a few. We, in the medical profession, simply manage those conditions, and people go on living full and happy lives. Herpes is exactly like that. You can treat it and live with it, even though you wish you didn't have it and that it would go away. And compared to HIV, diabetes, or hypertension, the physical impact of genital herpes is *far* less significant. The trick is getting your head in the right place about herpes. We'll discuss those emotional issues in chapter 8.

5. Can I give genital herpes to my children or roommates? No. Again, herpes is a sexually transmitted infection. It requires direct contact with the genital area to pass it from one person to another. (Sex toys are the small exception to this rule.) There isn't any risk of infecting children who live in your home. Kids aren't going to get herpes by touching your dirty laundry or sleeping in your bed. I do suggest that people use their own towels and washcloths, because these items can stay warm and moist for a while, and those are the conditions viruses love most. Having said that, there are no documented cases of anyone ever getting herpes from a towel. Roommates don't need to worry about getting herpes from couch cushions or from sharing kitchen utensils or bathtubs. Questions about nonsexual transmission in the home are very common, but just remember these three little words: "skin to skin" (which is also "mucous membrane to mucous membrane"). That's how herpes is passed from one person to another.

6. What's the best treatment strategy for my herpes?

That decision depends entirely on your social and sexual situation, and your feelings about herpes outbreaks. If you want to reduce the risk of passing herpes to someone else, taking preventive medicine every day will help. And if you're bothered by outbreaks, daily therapy will help with that too. If your partner also has herpes, and you aren't having frequent outbreaks, then maybe taking medicine only during outbreaks is enough for you. And, if you don't want to take medicine at all, you don't have to. Herpes isn't like a bacterial infection, which requires taking antibiotics to keep it from getting worse. With herpes, you take medicine to relieve symptoms or reduce the risk of passing the virus to someone else, not to permanently get rid of your herpes infection. In chapter 6, we'll talk more about choosing a treatment plan that's best for you. And it's good to remember that this choice isn't permanent: treatment decisions can be flexible and change if your situation changes.

7. How do I know if I really have herpes?

There are excellent tests available now for herpes, and they're much better than what we had only a few years ago. In the past, you had to have a herpes symptom present to make a diagnosis, but now there are blood antibody tests that detect herpes infection even if you've never had a symptom. And the swab tests that we have now are up to four times more sensitive than the older culture-style swab tests. Finding out that you have herpes through one of these tests is a double-edged sword. The bad news is that you find out you have herpes, but the good news is that you now know you have herpes and can manage it—whereas, if you didn't know you had it, you could do nothing about it. In chapter 4, we'll talk a lot more about diagnosing herpes, and also about misdiagnosis, which is a much more common problem than you might think.

8. Who gave me herpes, and how long have I had it?

Sometimes these two questions can be answered, but more often they can't. If you've only had one sex partner in your life and you now have herpes, you know where you got it—either from intercourse with that person or by receiving oral sex from him or her. If you've had more than one partner, it's going to be tougher to sort out. Let's say you get a new sore in the genital area, and you've never had one before. You get a swab test from the sore, and it comes back positive for *HSV 2* (*herpes simplex virus type 2*). During the same visit, you get a blood antibody test done for HSV 2, and it comes back negative. So you have HSV 2 in the sore, but you don't have any HSV 2 antibodies in your blood. You don't have the antibody, because the infection is brand new and not enough time has gone by for your body to make it. That means it's a new infection that you recently acquired. A positive IgG antibody test (a specific kind of blood test that we will talk about in great detail in chapter 4) combined with a positive swab test means that the infection has been present for at least a week or perhaps twenty years; with this combination, you can't know how long you've been infected.

Timing is important though. Fifty percent of people will make the antibody within three weeks of infection (Ashley-Morrow, Krantz, and Wald 2003), so if you're going to try to nail down new infection versus old, the tests have to happen fairly quickly after the first symptoms show up. But getting both tests at the same time is really the only way to know if the infection is new or old, and, perhaps, who gave it to you. We'll discuss all this and more in chapter 4.

9. Can I still have children? Definitely! Since almost one out of five American adults already has HSV 2 infection (Xu et al. 2006), it's apparent that many women are safely having babies despite having herpes. And the female partners of men with herpes are getting pregnant and having healthy babies too. The key to infected parents having a healthy baby is twofold: First, women and their partners need to know the herpes status of everyone involved. If a father has herpes but doesn't know it, he can unknowingly infect his female partner, and if that happens late in pregnancy, that's a very bad thing. A pregnant woman who gets herpes may not know about it and won't be taking the necessary precautions to protect her baby at delivery. Second, women need an obstetric provider who knows how to manage genital herpes or the risk of transmitting herpes to the baby during delivery. If a woman already has genital herpes and knows it, the risk of her giving it to her baby is very small indeed! We'll talk more about this in chapter 5.

10. Will my life ever be the same again? Though this may not be the first question people ask, it's the one that's at the heart of concerns about herpes. Babies, sex, blame, transmission, and symptoms—all of those concerns require that you think about herpes and deal with it. It really can't be ignored, so in that sense, yes, your life will be changed. But if you were to develop diabetes, you'd need to change your diet, take medicine, and track your blood sugars. You wouldn't, however, be a different person at the core of yourself. Yet somehow, maybe because you're dealing with a sexually transmitted disease, concern about this is greater when dealing with herpes. You might wonder, "Will people accept me the way I am? Will I be as happy as I was before this diagnosis? Will people think less of me? Will I live in fear of people discovering I have herpes?" It's good to know that three detailed studies have determined that most everyone who's newly diagnosed with herpes gets back to his or her former psychological functioning level within six months (Miyai et al. 2004). Yes, you have a virus in the genital area, but you're not really any different inside—unless, of course, you somehow let this virus define who you are. I'm going to try hard in chapter 8 to give you the tools to deal with the emotional concerns you might have about herpes.

So there are the top ten questions and ten very short answers. Did you find your question on the list? You'll see much more detail in the chapters to come. So let's dive in and meet the "Herpes Family." You might not want this family living in your "neighborhood," but you're about to learn that they already live in almost all "neighborhoods"!

Chapter 2

The Herpes Family of Viruses: Getting to Know the Whole Clan

Herpes is certainly not the first virus you've ever encountered, but you may not have thought much about viruses until now. You probably know that a virus causes the common cold, and you may have been told that a virus causes some of those twenty-four-hour upset-stomach episodes you dread. You've probably heard that bird flu is caused by a virus and so is the regular winter upper-respiratory flu. You may know that hepatitis is caused by a group of different viruses with names like A, B, and C. And now you've met one of the herpes viruses—up close and personal.

When you hear the word "herpes," you have something specific in mind: the genital or oral (or both) infection you have. But the medical term *herpes virus* refers to a group of eight different viruses that all share similar characteristics. The genital herpes you have is caused by just one of those eight. Having trouble getting your mind around the virus-group idea? Think about it this easy way. We use the term "dog" to describe a group of animals that have tails and wet noses, chase cats, and require housebreaking. Some are hounds, some are bulldogs, and some are Chihuahuas—and some are large, and some are small—but they all fall under the category of "dog."

Similarly, these eight viruses all fall under the name "herpes," but they're all slightly different from each other. Normally, I don't spend a lot of time talking about the basic science of herpes viruses. It's just not all that interesting to people who aren't scientists or researchers. But there's some confusion between these viruses when it comes to diagnosis, symptoms, and treatment, so I want you to be clear about which virus you have so that you can manage it appropriately. For example, is that rash on your hip a reactivation of the chicken pox you had as a child, or is it herpes simplex? Can it be transmitted to others through sex or from coughing? Is the tiredness and sore throat you're feeling due to Epstein-Barr virus or to strep throat? If you get pregnant, is your baby more at risk from herpes simplex or another herpes virus, cytomegalovirus? Because of questions like these, I'll walk you through this "dog show" to minimize the confusion. If, after reading this, you're still confused about which virus you have, ask your health care provider. You'll at least be better equipped with your own information and ready to ask good questions.

THE FAMILY OF EIGHT

The eight herpes viruses that infect people share one really big thing in common: once you get them, they live in your body for the rest of your life. And if that weren't true, genital herpes wouldn't be a big deal at all, would it? You'd take some pills, it would go away, and you'd feel much relieved. Let's look briefly at the eight viruses now. You'll see where your genital virus fits in and how it's different from the others that share its name.

For each virus, I'll give you the medical name, the abbreviation, the disease or diseases it causes, the potential complications, how the virus is transmitted, the available treatments, and whether or not there's vaccine to prevent it.

Herpes Simplex Virus Type 1

Abbreviation: HSV 1

Diseases: Oral (cold sores) and genital herpes, herpes of the eye

Complications: Blindness (rare), neonatal herpes (rare), encephalitis (rare), probably Bell's palsy (uncommon), recurrent aseptic meningitis

Transmitted: Skin-to-skin contact (kissing, oral sex, vaginal and anal intercourse, naked genital-to-genital rubbing)

Treatment: Antiviral medicines

Vaccine: No

Herpes Simplex Virus Type 2

Abbreviation: HSV 2

Diseases: The more common form of genital herpes, herpes of the eye (uncommon), oral herpes (rare)

Complications: Neonatal herpes (rare), encephalitis (rare), recurrent aseptic meningitis

Transmitted: Skin-to-skin contact (kissing, oral sex, vaginal and anal intercourse, naked genital-to-genital rubbing, from mother to baby during birth)

Treatment: Antiviral medicines

Vaccine: In clinical trials

Varicella-Zoster Virus

Abbreviation: VZV

Diseases: Chicken pox and then shingles later in life when reactivated (also known as *herpes zoster*)

Complications: Severe illness (like pneumonia, hepatitis, or encephalitis) in some who get chicken pox, and postherpetic neuralgia in some older adults who get shingles.

Transmitted: Airborne droplets from breathing and coughing, skin-to-skin contact

Treatment: Antiviral medicines

Vaccine: For chicken pox, Varivax (varicella virus vaccine) should be given at age 1, and a booster between ages 4 and 6. Adults and teens who've had only one dose should also get a booster. There's a related vaccine for shingles, Zostavax (herpes zoster vaccine, live attenuated), that's FDA approved for people aged 60 and older. It's a single-dose vaccine that's often available at local pharmacies, as flu shots are, as well as from your health care provider.

Epstein-Barr Virus

Abbreviation: EBV

Diseases: Mononucleosis (also known as mono, or "the kissing disease")

Complications: Most AIDS-associated lymphomas, other lymphomas, and some nasopharyngeal carcinomas

Transmitted: Airborne droplets, kissing

Treatment: Not required for most common conditions

Vaccine: No

Cytomegalovirus

Abbreviation: CMV

Diseases: Usually no disease associated with infection; occasionally mononucleosis

Complications: Women who get newly infected during pregnancy can bear children with a variety of problems. People whose immune systems aren't functioning well, such as those who have HIV, are transplant patients, or are undergoing chemotherapy, can have a reactivation of this virus and experience a variety of problems, some severe, related to CMV infection.

Transmitted: Airborne, maternal-fetal intrauterine infection, blood products, transplanted organs

Treatment: Antiviral medicines

Vaccine: In clinical trials

Human Herpes Virus 6

Abbreviation: HHV 6

Diseases: Roseola in infants, characterized by high fever, pea-shaped bumps at the back of the head, and body rashes

Complications: Encephalitis (rare)

Transmitted: Airborne

Treatment: None

Vaccine: No

Human Herpes Virus 7

Abbreviation: HHV 7

Diseases: Body rash in children

Complications: Usually none

Transmitted: Airborne

Treatment: None

Vaccine: No

Human Herpes Virus 8 (or Kaposi's Sarcoma)

Abbreviations: HHV 8 or KSHV

Disease: Blood-vessel associated cancers, purplish-red skin lesions, rare types of lymphoma

Complications: The spreading of the above diseases throughout the whole body

Transmitted: Unknown

Treatment: Antiretroviral therapy for AIDS-associated KSHV

Vaccine: No

More About Varicella-Zoster Virus

Let's talk a little more about varicella-zoster virus (VZV), because it's the one that most often gets confused with herpes simplex virus. As you read above, varicella-zoster virus causes chicken pox. Once the chicken pox rash is gone, VZV becomes "latent" in your body, meaning that it goes to sleep but doesn't actually go away. Shingles (herpes zoster) is a reactivation or a reawakening of the chicken pox virus. Shingles occurs mostly in older people, because as we age, we get farther and farther away from our original case of chicken pox, and our immune response to VZV gets weaker and weaker. Shingles appears as a painful, blistery rash that affects only one side of the body. The VZV usually travels along a single nerve, and the rash runs from the middle of the body in the front, around the side to the middle in the back, or vice versa. Sometimes the rash doesn't go all the way around; it might just appear on the side of the chest or on one hip, for example. But shingles rarely crosses an imaginary line that runs down the middle of the body. People often get strange sensations in the skin before the blistery rash appears: tingling, irritation, itching, prickling, skin sensitivity, and even tenderness or a bruised feeling. Then the blistery rash appears. Unfortunately, some people continue to feel the pain of shingles for months or even years after the rash has disappeared. This ongoing pain is called *postherpetic neuralgia* (*PHN*), and it can be very difficult for those who have it. Treatment options for PHN are limited, and the pain can be life changing. Prevention of PHN is the main reason for getting the shingles vaccination, Zostavax. If you are sixty or older, please get this important vaccine.

Laypeople and even clinicians sometimes get herpes simplex and herpes zoster (shingles) mixed up. People with herpes simplex virus can mistakenly be told they have shingles, and vice versa. Perhaps this has happened to you. At some point, maybe you were told you had shingles on your hip, and now, years later, you're diagnosed with genital herpes, and you have no idea where it came from! It's not really surprising that these two infections get mixed up. They both can cause a blistery rash. Both of the rashes can occur in the area from waist to midthigh (though the majority of shingles cases shows up on the chest or abdomen). Both can be painful and perceived as a change in nerve and skin sensations. But there's a key, essential difference: shingles rarely recurs. Only about 3 percent of people who get it the first time ever get it again, and almost no one gets it a third time (Gnann Jr. and Whitley 2002). On the other hand, genital HSV 2 infection recurs in almost everyone (whether they recognize it or not), and not infrequently. The other obvious difference is that there's varicella-zoster virus in the blisters of one rash and herpes simplex virus in the blisters of the other. A swab sample gathered from the rash and sent to a laboratory can accurately sort out VZV from HSV infection. We'll talk more about VZV getting confused with HSV in chapter 4. For now, the thing to remember is this: if a rash is recurring, think herpes simplex virus and not varicella-zoster virus.

But wait—the plot thickens! Sometimes clinicians tell people who have suspicious rashes on their hips or buttocks that they have herpes zoster, even though the clinicians actually suspect or even *know* that their patients have herpes simplex.

As time has passed and I've interacted with more and more clinicians around the country, I've discovered that this strategy is more common than I'd ever imagined. It isn't done maliciously and is intended to protect patients from what's believed to be "really bad news," and perhaps also to avoid "opening the can of worms" a herpes diagnosis requires. Some of those clinicians even consider my personal approach of correctly diagnosing as many HSV 2-infected people as possible to be intentionally harmful and insensitive to the feelings of perfectly nice people. It's always interesting how things look from another perspective, isn't it?

While it's true that no one yearns to hear a herpes diagnosis, if you don't know you have it, you simply can't manage it effectively. The patients of a medical practice who are told they have recurrent shingles but really have genital herpes get cheated out of knowing the truth about their physical conditions. Though the news of genital herpes is upsetting to many people, we simply can't let social stigma guide medical practice. At least that's how I see it.

Before we move to an in-depth discussion of the "big two," HSV 1 and 2, let me share with you the most common questions I'm asked about VZV:

Commonly Asked Questions About VZV

I had chicken pox as a child. Could that be the reason why my HSV 2 antibody test looks positive? I've never had any symptoms of genital herpes. No. The IgG type-specific herpes simplex virus antibody tests can accurately distinguish between VZV and HSV. However, the less accurate IgM tests may not be able to tell the difference. One of the reasons I tell people never to get IgM testing done for herpes is the possibility of what's called "cross-reactivity" between other herpes viruses and herpes simplex in that test. That means that one virus shows up looking like another. If you don't know what type of testing you had done, check and see. Most people who've had a positive TgG HSV antibody test insisted before they were tested that they couldn't possibly have genital herpes, but they really do, and they can infect others. Look for more information about the best available tests in chapter 4.

Can the vaccines for chicken pox and zoster help protect me from getting herpes or treat the herpes that I already have? No, they can't. Varivax and Zostavax vaccines are specifically designed to protect only against VZV, not herpes simplex, and they won't reduce the chance of getting genital or oral herpes, nor will they treat an existing infection.

My doctor told me I have recurrent shingles on my buttocks. I get it about four times a year. Why would you tell me it could be genital herpes instead? I'm not a promiscuous person, and I've had the same partner for five years. Couldn't I just be the exception to the rule that shingles doesn't recur? Shingles rarely recurs even once in the healthy adult. And since you're having this rash on your hip about four times a year, I have real concerns about the accuracy of your shingles diagnosis. The next time you get this blistery rash, have a swab test done for herpes simplex and also for varicella-zoster virus when the rash is just starting. Or just have a type-specific antibody test for HSV 2 done at any time.

I'm thirty years old. I was diagnosed with HSV 2 by a PCR swab test from a genital sore. I get pain down the back of my leg from time to time, and I've read a lot about postherpetic neuralgia from shingles. Does the pain in my leg mean I have shingles also, or could I have this pain from genital herpes? My guess is that the pain relates more to genital herpes than shingles, but it could relate to neither. At thirty, I wouldn't expect you to have shingles, though it's possible. You could have a spinal-disk problem or something completely unrelated that's causing the pain. Some people with genital herpes do get pain in the back of the leg as the virus becomes more active in that nerve group, and this can be one of a group of symptoms called *prodrome* that signal the beginning of an outbreak. Sometimes the pain even goes down into the foot. PHN from shingles tends to be persistent rather than intermittent.

I'm forty-five years old, and I've never had chicken pox. My partner has genital herpes, and now I'm worried that if I get herpes, I could also get chicken pox. Should I be worried? No, you don't need to be worried about getting chicken pox from someone who has herpes. These viruses are in the same family, but you don't get one virus from the other. By the way, at your age, almost everyone in the United States has had chicken pox infection (Gnann Jr. and Whitley 2002). You probably had a minor case and just missed it. There's a blood test to find out.

I'm fifty-eight years old, I have genital herpes, and I bought this book to learn more about my disease, but the discussion about shingles has piqued my interest. My mother had a very bad case of shingles and PHN, and I'd certainly like to avoid that. Am I too young for the shingles vaccine? I've got very good insurance coverage for this kind of thing. No, you aren't too young to get the vaccine, but you're too young for insurance to pay for it. For now, Zostavax is FDA approved for people aged sixty and over. It works just fine for people a little younger, but the FDA-approval studies were done on a specific population of people over sixty, and for now, most insurance only covers the vaccine based on the FDA approval. That could change if new studies show benefit in a younger population. You could wait a year and get the vaccine, or you could get it earlier and pay for it yourself.

Now that we've talked about the other herpes viruses, let's go into more detail about HSV 1 and HSV 2 infections.

Herpes Simplex Virus Type 1 (HSV 1)

Disease it causes: HSV 1 causes the majority of recurrent cold sores (also called fever blisters) that show up on the lips, nose, chin, and other parts of the face. These sores most often start out as small water blisters that open, form a crust, and then heal. Cold sores normally recur two to three times per year, and they got their name because they sometimes show up when people have another illness (like the common cold) at the same time. However, most HSV 1 oral infections don't show up with clear symptoms or have symptoms that go unrecognized, so many people who are infected don't know it. People can "give off" herpes simplex virus type 1 or 2 when they have symptoms but aren't aware of them. This process of giving off the virus from the body is called *shedding*. It's like what a cat or dog does with hair, but with herpes, much of the time you can't see shedding happening, no matter how well you "know" your body, or how carefully or frequently you check. Shedding that happens when no symptoms are present is called *asymptomatic viral shedding*.

HSV 1 also causes the majority of herpes of the eye, also called *ocular herpes* or *herpes keratitis*. Sometimes, the virus travels along the top branch of the nerve that provides nerve sensation to the face and the eyes. Sometimes a person touches a first-infection cold sore and then touches an eye, which can transfer the infection from the mouth to the eye. This is called *autoinoculation*, which means that you yourself move a virus from one part of your body to another, but this normally happens only during first-episode infections, before an immune response has been established. That immune response keeps you from getting new herpes outbreaks on other parts of your body. However it gets there, herpes of the eye is not a good thing to have, but thankfully, it isn't all that common and is very treatable (though not curable presently). However, treatment is essential to avoid damage to the cornea of the eye. For managing herpes of the eye, it's a very good idea to consult a physician who specializes in eye diseases (opthalmologist).

This can be shocking news for some, but HSV 1 can also cause genital herpes. In fact, HSV 1 now accounts for almost 40 percent of new genital herpes infections in the United States. In teens and college students, HSV 1 accounts for even more new herpes cases than HSV 2, probably because of the popularity of oral sex among young people (Roberts, Pfister, and Spear 2003). In certain other countries, more than half of genital herpes is now HSV 1 rather than HSV 2 (Malkin 2004). Here are some things that people with genital HSV 1 infection should know:

- HSV 1 genital infection is often a result of mouth-to-genital transmission. This can happen in couples who've never before had sex with anyone but each other.

- This kind of transmission can happen whether cold sores are present or not.

- Genital HSV 1 outbreaks recur infrequently, about once every other year or less (Engelberg et al. 2003; Lafferty et al. 1987).

- Almost half the people infected with genital HSV 1 have no recurrences at all (Lafferty et al. 1987).

- HSV 1 in the genital area gives off the virus from the body (or sheds) on average about five days out of a hundred. That means that during an average month, you'd give off the virus on about one or two days. Remember that a lot of this shedding happens without any symptoms.

- Though HSV 1 is causing many *new* genital herpes cases, HSV 2 is the main culprit for *recurrent* outbreaks. Over 90 percent of recurrent genital herpes is due to HSV 2; HSV 1 recurs genitally far less often (Malkin 2004).

Oral outbreak "triggers": Researchers don't know what triggers an outbreak of herpes, but one thing that has been scientifically proven to trigger cold sores is sunlight. If you get cold sores, you've probably noticed that when you spend a day at the beach or out on the snow in bright sun, you may pay a price a few days later with a cold sore. Lip balms that contain a high-SPF sunscreen may reduce the number of fever blisters that you get. Another trigger is trauma, not necessarily the car-accident variety but more the facial-surgery kind. If you go to a plastic surgeon to have your lips plumped or your face lifted even just a little, you'll probably be asked if you have a history of cold sores. If you do, you'll probably be advised to take antiviral therapy for a week or so before the procedure so that when they jostle your facial nerves during the surgery, the recovery won't be complicated by a cold sore. Other triggers that aren't well documented but are often reported by people are stress, lack of sleep, changing time zones, eating spicy food, and the prolonged or rough giving of oral sex.

Who's infected? As of this writing, about 56 percent of people in the United States over the age of fourteen have HSV 1 infection (Xu et al. 2006). We don't know from blood antibody tests exactly who has oral herpes and who has genital herpes. We only know that 56 percent of the adult population has the antibody to HSV 1, so they're infected with it somewhere on their bodies. Furthermore, a positive antibody test means that a person is infectious to others.

Herpes Simplex Virus Type 2 (HSV 2)

Who has HSV 2? HSV 2 infects lots of different people in the United States. The table below contains data telling us who's infected by age, gender, race, and other factors, like level of education and number of sexual partners in a lifetime. Please note that the ethnic categories were self-reported as shown. Look over the table to see where you fit in.

Herpes Simplex Virus Type 2
Seroprevalence 1999–2004

Overall HSV 2 seroprevalence	17%
All males aged 14–19	1%
All males aged 20–29	6%
All males aged 30–39	15%
All males aged 40–49	19%
All females aged 14–19	2%
All females aged 20–29	16%
All females aged 30–39	30%
All females aged 40–49	34%
Non-Hispanic whites aged 14–19	1%
Non-Hispanic whites aged 20–29	6%
Non-Hispanic whites aged 30–39	18%
Non-Hispanic whites age 40–49	21%
Non-Hispanic blacks aged 14–19	50%
Non-Hispanic blacks aged 20–29	35%
Non-Hispanic blacks aged 30–39	54%
Non-Hispanic blacks aged 40–49	56%
Mexican Americans aged 14–19	1%
Mexican Americans aged 20–29	8%
Mexican Americans aged 30–39	14%

Mexican Americans aged 40–49	25%
Never married	10%
Living with partner	25%
Married	17%
Divorced	36%
Separated	35%
Widowed	47%
< High-school education	16%
> or = High-school education	18%
First sexual encounter < or = age 17	21%
First sexual encounter > or = age 18	14%
0 lifetime sexual partners	2%
1 lifetime sexual partner	4%
2–4 lifetime sexual partners	13%
5–9 lifetime sexual partners	21%
10–49 lifetime sexual partners	27%
> or = 50 lifetime sexual partners	40%

Source: Data adapted with permission from Xu et al. 2006. Copyright © 2006 American Medical Association. All rights reserved.

Disease it causes: HSV 2 is the virus more commonly associated with genital herpes. The symptoms of genital herpes vary greatly from person to person and, to some degree, from outbreak to outbreak. I'm reluctant to describe a "typical" first outbreak or a "typical" recurrence, because there's so much variation in how they appear. There's an incorrect idea floating around out there that every first infection with herpes is severe, but often it's not. A first infection with either HSV 1 or 2 can produce multiple painful sores, a single one that's hardly noticeable, or no symptoms at all. Symptoms of genital herpes may include:

- Blisters
- Sores

- Itchy areas

- Skin cracks

- Skin fissures

- Skin ulcers

- Irritated areas

- Areas that look as if the skin has been rubbed off

- Pain during urination (from lesions inside the urethra in men and women)

- Watery discharge from the penis or vagina

- Pain down the leg (neuralgia) when the virus becomes active on the nerve

The following charts show the symptoms people have with primary and recurrent infection (Corey 1988). As you'll see in these charts, in general, people with first-episode infection have more symptoms than those having recurrences.

CHARACTERISTICS OF PEOPLE WITH PRIMARY HSV 2 INFECTION

	Men	Women
Fever, malaise, headache	39%	68%
Pain at site of outbreak	95%	99%
Duration of pain	11 days	12 days
Urethral or vaginal discharge	27%	85%
Duration of discharge	6 days	13 days
Swollen lymph nodes	80%	81%
Painful urination	44%	83%

CHARACTERISTICS OF PEOPLE HAVING RECURRENT GENITAL HERPES EPISODES

	Men	Women
Prodromal symptoms	53%	43%
Lesional pain	67%	88%
Itching of lesions	85%	87%
Painful urination	9%	27%
Swollen lymph nodes	23%	31%
Urethral or vaginal discharge	4%	45%
Average duration of pain	4 days	6 days

Some people experience nongenital symptoms with their herpes, such as headache, sensitivity to light, swollen lymph nodes, low-grade fever, nerve pain in the leg, or (for oral herpes) pain in the face. Here are some things that people infected with genital HSV 2 should know:

- HSV 2 is almost always transmitted from the genitals of one person to the genitals of another.

- HSV 2 virus is shed from the genitals quite often, on average around 20 percent of the time, with some studies reporting up to 40 percent of days, some as low as 4 percent of days (Sacks et al. 2004), and this often happens when no symptoms are present (as mentioned earlier, known as "asymptomatic shedding"). This means that if a person swabs his or her genitals at home for 100 days, virus might be recovered from those swabs on 20 to 40 of the 100 days the swabbing is done.

- Even if you've never had any symptoms but test positive on an antibody test for HSV 2, you have the virus and can pass it to others (Wald et al. 2000).

- People with HSV 2 typically have three to five recurrences per year, but about 20 percent of people with HSV 2 have more than ten recurrences per year (Benedetti, Corey, and Ashley 1994). There's a lot of variation in how people experience outbreaks.

- Over time, you'll have fewer recurrences, but shedding, the giving off of virus from your body with or without symptoms, never goes away. You should assume that your herpes is a lifelong infection, regardless of whether or not you have symptoms.

WHAT HERPES ISN'T

It might be helpful to talk about what symptoms are *not* herpes. It's not a skin growth that sticks out from the body and stays around for quite a while. It's not a skin bump with a little dot in the center that has a hard, white center. It's not a condition where bumps show up all over your body. It's not a flat, red, blanket-like rash that spreads around the thigh or groin. Herpes doesn't cause a fishy odor or a clumpy white discharge that smells like bread. It most often doesn't cause a thick, yellow discharge from the end of the penis that requires you to put toilet paper in your undershorts. And it's not something you experience every day. Herpes symptoms come and go intermittently. It's also not the end of the world, even though on some days it might feel like that.

WHERE DOES HERPES SHOW UP?

HSV 2 can cause symptoms anywhere in the boxer-shorts area. That's because the virus lives in a group of nerves at the base of the spine called the *sacral ganglia*. This group of nerves supplies sensation to the entire pelvic area, not just the genitals, so outbreaks of genital herpes can appear on the buttocks, hip, thigh, lower abdomen, anus, gluteal cleft (that would be the "plumber's crack" area), and, of course, on the genitals. Outbreaks are not limited to the site where you were first infected with the virus. For example, you might get outbreaks around the anus, but that doesn't necessarily mean that you first got herpes from anal sex. The virus can travel along any nerve to get to the surface of the skin, not just the nerve it came in on. I tell my patients that there are lots of ways to get from New York to Seattle: you can take the interstates directly, or you can take the back roads and other highways and still get there. Herpes is the same. It can go back out the way it came in, or it can follow a different nerve in the same nerve group and end up somewhere else in the boxer-shorts area. And locations can vary from outbreak to outbreak. Some people always have recurrences in the same location, and other people have outbreaks that move. But if your outbreaks move, don't assume that *you're* doing anything to move them. The virus just picks a different nerve on which to travel. And no, we don't know why its travel plans change. So far, it's managed to keep that a secret.

Outbreak triggers: There are no well-documented triggers for genital herpes outbreaks, but many possibilities have been discussed: friction from sexual contact (again, a form of "trauma"), stress, illness, lack of sleep, specific foods, and menstrual periods. The only one that's been scientifically proven to be a trigger is extended periods of stress lasting more than two weeks, and prolonged stress is linked to only a very slight increase in the likelihood of having an outbreak (Rein 2000; Cohen et al. 1999). Just as with oral herpes, there are some generally accepted outside-induced triggers; for example, exposure to ultraviolet light (so keep that swimsuit bottom on!) and undergoing lower-abdominal or back surgery could result in an outbreak (because the nerves get traumatized in that area). Also, if anything suppresses your immune response, you may be more vulnerable to an outbreak. This would include things like taking steroids for an asthma attack, being on cancer chemotherapy, or having advanced HIV disease.

Who's infected? Almost 1 in 5 people in the United States over the age of fourteen has HSV 2 infection (Xu et al. 2006). That means, for example, that 20 of the 100 senators in Congress are likely to have genital herpes (though, of those, probably only 2 know they have it). The more sex partners you have, the more likely you are to have herpes. It's just a matter of statistics: more partners means there's a greater chance that someone you had sex with had herpes. But don't forget: you can get herpes from a single sex partner too. You're more likely to have HSV 2 if you're female, because if you're the "receiving" partner during intercourse (meaning there's a penis rubbing virus into your vaginal mucous membranes), transmission is simply easier and more "efficient." In the

United States, if you're an African American over the age of fourteen, there's about a 50 percent chance that you have HSV 2 infection (Xu et al. 2006). We're not totally clear as to why that's true, but more than one large study has shown it to be the case.

These two types of herpes virus have what we call "site preferences." HSV 1 "prefers" the oral area, meaning that it recurs more there and sheds virus from there more often, but can infect and recur in the genital area. HSV 2, on the other hand, strongly prefers the genital area and only infrequently affects the oral area. It's possible, of course, to give oral sex to and have intercourse with the same person and get infected at both locations with the same virus at the same time. About 10 percent of people diagnosed with primary (no previous infection with HSV 1 or 2) genital herpes can also have the same type of virus isolated from the oral area (Corey 1988). The following chart shows how approximately much each virus sheds in the oral and genital area. These numbers come from studies in which people swabbed their genitals or mouths every day at home to look for viral shedding (Miller and Danaher 2008). Typically people swabbed once a day, but in recent studies, Dr. Anna Wald (Mark et al. 2008), at the University of Washington, had people swabbing four times per day, because she wondered whether we were missing very short-term outbreaks with once-a-day swabbing. She found significantly more shedding with four swabs per day and also discovered that many shedding episodes lasted less than twelve hours. I guess you could say, the more we look for shedding, the more we find. This means that the virus is "on" more often than we previously thought, which explains why people often pass the virus on to others even though they don't have any symptoms.

Herpes Shedding

HSV 2 genital shedding	15–25% of days
HSV 1 oral shedding	6–33% of days
HSV 1 genital shedding	5% of days
HSV 2 oral shedding	1% of days

COMMON QUESTIONS ABOUT HSV 1 AND 2

I get recurrent cold sores that have swab-tested positive for HSV 1. If I give my partner oral sex and he gets genital herpes from my mouth, will his genital herpes turn into type 2 because it's in his genital area? No, the virus is what it is regardless of where it is. If a gay man walks into a straight bar, he doesn't become straight. He's still gay even if he's in a straight bar for a visit. The same is true with this virus (except that with a bar visit, you can leave and this virus doesn't). It is what its DNA says it is, and being someplace other than its preferred location doesn't change that. It will still be HSV 1 in the genital area, and it will never change into HSV 2.

I got a rash on my thigh, which I thought was poison oak, but my doctor said his swab test indicates it's genital herpes type 2. I'm into kind of kinky stuff sometimes, but I never have thigh sex (whatever that is). How could this be? Remember the boxer-shorts description? Genital herpes infects that group of nerves that supplies sensation to the area that might be typically covered by a pair of boxer shorts, and your thigh is in that area. The virus you got through a sexual encounter simply decided to resurface on your thigh. You may have missed the first genital outbreak or figured that your symptoms were due to something other than herpes, like jock itch, friction burn, or a zipper pinch. Do you remember anything like that happening? It may have been your initial outbreak of herpes.

I swear that stress causes me to have outbreaks. And then I get stressed out about being stressed! This feels like a vicious cycle. Maybe for you, it's true that stress is associated with your outbreaks. But research doesn't back that up for the general public. Good studies have been done on stress in particular, and they don't find a correlation between short-term stressful events and herpes outbreaks (Rand et al. 1990). It might help to look at it this way: instead of getting a herpes outbreak and looking *backward* to see if you were stressed, you might want to make a note on a calendar every time you feel stress, and then watch to see whether or not you get an outbreak. Many people get "stressed out about being stressed," and that situation just isn't very helpful. I would suggest that you consider a meditation class or see a therapist who can help you to think differently about stress. If you believe that stress is making your herpes worse, then you'll fear having stress in your life. Everyone, however, has unavoidable stress in his or her life, and it's pointless to try to avoid stress altogether. Perhaps a better strategy is to learn to cope with stress more effectively. And keep that calendar. I think you might be surprised at how often you have stressful events in your life that aren't followed by a herpes outbreak.

I have HSV 2 genitally, and my new sexual partner has been diagnosed with HSV 1 genitally. What should we do about our sexual relationship? Are we both vulnerable to getting each other's herpes? You're very unlikely to get her HSV 1, since HSV 2 appears to offer protection against most HSV 1. However, she's vulnerable to your HSV 2. You two should behave as though she's uninfected with genital herpes, and do what you can to avoid transmission of the HSV 2, if that's your desire. Some research indicates that long-term HSV 2–negative partners of people who have HSV 2 have an immune response to the virus that isn't equivalent to infection but may confer some protection against infection (Posavad et al. 2003).

I'm a straight guy, but I get all my herpes outbreaks around my anus. I swear I've never had any sexual contact there with anyone, and I'm so embarrassed and worried about what my clinician will think when I show up with these ulcers. Will everyone talk about me when I leave the office? Remember what I said about traveling from New York to Seattle, that there are lots of different ways you can go? Well, your HSV 2 basically took the shortest path to get to the surface of the skin. If the virus hangs out at the base of the spine and you get your outbreaks around the anus, that's probably the quickest way the virus can get to the surface of the skin. Draw an imaginary line in your head from your tailbone to your anus and compare the distance to your penis. Are you getting the picture? People in professional health care understand this, but even if they don't, do you really need their approval and for them to believe that your sex partners are exclusively female? Probably not, in most cases. Read more about this "approval" business in chapter 8, on psychological adjustment.

Chapter 3

Transmission: What You Wish You Had Known Sooner

Now, I'd like to talk about the possibility of giving genital herpes to other people: how it happens, how it doesn't, how likely it is, what you can to do to reduce the risk, how effective these strategies really are, and, finally, how to come to terms with sex while living with genital herpes.

If herpes were a disease that you had all to yourself that couldn't be given to others, it would be quite a different thing, wouldn't it? You'd deal with outbreaks as they came up, and that would be it. But the fact that it's sexually transmissible makes it more difficult and stigmatized. Our society has some well-defined negative views about STIs, as you may have noticed. And no one is eager to pass herpes on to someone else. In fact, the biggest fear of most people with genital herpes is giving it to someone else.

It's pretty easy to slip into thinking of yourself as a virus waiting to be shared rather than a person with many fine qualities who simply has a virus with the potential to be shared. Do you appreciate that important difference? So let's first talk about the language we'll use to discuss this topic. I personally don't like the term "spread" as it relates to herpes. "Spread" is something you do with mayonnaise, and it has an almost intentional quality when applied to herpes. Instead, I'll use the terms "transmit," "give," "pass," or "infect" to describe the mechanism of "sharing" this virus with someone else.

GIVING GENITAL HERPES TO OTHERS

Genital herpes is transmitted from one person to another through some kind of sexual contact—period. Most often, that's vaginal or anal intercourse. It's possible that a person with genital herpes could give it to a partner through other sexual activities. I'll list those, but please keep in mind that the risk of transmission is really low for the nongenital behavior; it just isn't zero. If you have genital herpes and someone gives you oral sex, he or she could get herpes on the mouth. Naked genital-to-genital rubbing, or "outercourse," could result in a genital infection in your partner. The degree of risk varies depending upon the kind of rubbing that happens, the amount of genital secretions present, how long you do it, and so on. The virus can also be transmitted through sex toys during a sexual encounter (but not from a vibrator that's been sitting in a nightstand drawer for days and then gets touched accidentally by your toddler).

How Herpes Is Not Transmitted

Herpes is not transmitted by using a public toilet seat, touching doorknobs, or from your doctor's speculum during your annual exam. It isn't transmitted from someone's giving you a lap dance while you're fully clothed, even if you have—uhhhh—"moisture" on your pants. That's right: the virus does not wick through clothing. It isn't transmitted by sharing a bar of soap or by sitting on the furniture of someone who has herpes. It isn't transmitted by mutual masturbation. It isn't transmitted while trying on swimsuits—but you're supposed to try those on wearing underwear anyway, remember? It isn't transmitted in swimming pools or hot tubs—unless you're having sex in there. And it certainly isn't transmitted to household members by ordinary social interactions like hugging or kissing, or holding your baby close to you.

How Does It Happen?

Even though we know how herpes is transmitted, there's no 100 percent foolproof way to keep from giving it to a sexual partner other than by abstaining from any sexual contact that involves parts of your body that are infected. It's good to start from that honest premise, because all the information you'll learn in this book about ways to reduce risk will empower you even more from that point on. I believe you'll be pleasantly surprised when you see the statistics about how low you can make your transmission potential.

The transmission of herpes from one partner to another happens when one person is infected and the other is not, and to that statement you'll rightly say, "Duh!" But the only way to really know whether or not someone has herpes is to take a test to determine herpes status. You simply can't assume that someone is uninfected, even if he or she says so, because almost 90 percent of people who already have HSV 2 don't know they're infected (Leone et al. 2004)! So just asking someone, "Do you have genital herpes?" will only produce the correct answer some-times. You (and your partner) have no way of knowing whether your partner's response is correct unless he or she gets tested. So it's absolutely essential that both partners have antibody testing done so that the real risk of transmission can be accurately determined. We'll discuss testing in detail in chapter 4.

What If You Both Have Herpes?

"Well," you might say, "I don't have all of my sex partners tested. I just assume they're vulnerable to getting herpes from me, so I take the most conservative precautions so that they don't become infected." That's an okay strategy in the short run, but it may not be the best in the long run. Just think about it. If both parties are already infected with the same type of genital herpes (for example, both have HSV 1, or both have HSV 2), transmission is no longer of any concern—*if* you know about it. The virus won't be passed back and forth during sex; you can't get again what you already have. There's actually a great freedom that can come from that situation. Sex can blossom whenever the mood strikes (taking into account acceptable social norms, of course). There's no need to worry about triggering outbreaks in each other or passing the virus back and forth. If the infection has been around for a few months, you needn't be too concerned about passing the virus to a new part of the body (like the mouth) through sexual activities, because that very rarely happens. Assuming that other STIs have been ruled out, there's no need for concern about using condoms (except for birth control), taking daily medicine to reduce the risk of transmission, or watching for outbreaks. You can go back to spontaneous sex, just the same as before infection. It's a done deal.

When Only One Partner Has Herpes

But let's change the scenario and say that you find out through correct testing that you're infected with genital herpes and your partner is not. In official medical language, you two are determined to be "discordant": one is infected; the other is not. And since two types of herpes exist, HSV 1 and 2, there are several different combinations and permutations that could apply to your particular situation.

You have only oral HSV 1; your partner has neither HSV 1 nor 2. If you have oral HSV 1 infection and give oral sex to your partner, who has neither HSV 1 nor 2, HSV 1 could be transferred from your mouth to your partner's genitals, resulting in genital HSV 1 infection. Remember, a cold sore doesn't need to be present for this to occur, but avoiding giving oral sex when you have a cold sore certainly makes sense. Kissing could also transmit the virus from your mouth to the mouth of your partner, and your partner could get a new oral infection (known as a fever blister or cold sore). If the kissing is a peck kind of kiss and there's no cold sore present, transmission is highly unlikely. Wet, passionate kissing is more likely to result in oral-to-oral transmission. But it's important to not get so afraid of transmitting herpes that you fear any intimacy; life is about balance, after all.

You have genital HSV 1, and your partner has neither HSV 1 nor 2. Remember from the herpes shedding chart in chapter 2 that genital HSV 1 doesn't shed very often, so the risk is low of transmitting it through either intercourse or receiving oral sex. It's all about how often your genital virus is shed—not just about which part of your partner's body is exposed to your virus. So the chance that you'll infect your partner with HSV 1 is small, not zero, and we don't have specific numbers on this risk. And if your partner is pregnant, all the "rules" change. We'll talk more about that in chapter 5.

You have HSV 2, and your partner doesn't. If you have HSV 2 and your partner doesn't, your partner is at risk of getting herpes, mostly through vaginal or anal intercourse. Remember, genital HSV 2 sheds fairly often from the genitals, perhaps an average of one in every five days, regardless of your outbreak frequency, so this is the most risky scenario. "Just how risky?" you ask.

Several studies have looked at herpes transmission rates in couples, and following is what we know if you're an infected male who has an uninfected female partner under these conditions:

- Your partner knows you have genital herpes.

- You don't have sex while recognized symptoms are present.

- You don't use condoms, or you use them inconsistently.

- You don't take daily antiviral therapy.

The transmission rate from male to female has been shown, in various studies, to be 7 percent or 16 percent or 31 percent in a year—perhaps, for argument's sake, let's say an average of about 10 percent per year (Corey et al. 2004; Bryson et al. 1993; Mertz et al. 1992). Some studies have found that if you already have HSV 1, you're slightly less likely to get HSV 2, but other studies have not identified any difference (Looker and Garnett 2005). What we do know from a large study in pregnant women is that if you have HSV 2, you're highly unlikely to get HSV 1 infection later (Brown et al. 1997). So what does a 10 percent per year risk mean? It means that of a hundred couples in this same situation (and who have sex only with each other), ten partners would get HSV 2 from their infected partners within one year.

If the situation were reversed, with the women infected with HSV 2 but not their male partners with the same other factors, about 4 percent of the women would transmit the virus to their partners within a year (Mertz et al. 1992). Unfortunately, we don't have studies that look at the frequency of herpes transmission in same-sex couples.

Statistics in Studies of HSV Transmission

The statistics mentioned above come from couples who participated in medical research studies. We strongly advised them to use condoms, and they became well educated during the course of the research project, so the involvement with researchers could very well have reduced the transmission rate. The couples all *knew* that one was infected and the other wasn't. In everyday life, this isn't usually the case. If 90 percent of people who have HSV 2 don't know it, then only about one in ten discordant couples is aware that herpes is part of their relationship. The study couples had been together long enough to decide to participate in the study, since you don't just meet someone in a bar and say, "Hi, my name's Linda. I have genital herpes. Would you like to do a research study with me?" Herpes often gets transmitted in the early days of relationships, perhaps because people have sex more frequently in that phase of the relationship, sexual encounters last longer or are more vigorous than later in the relationship, and those people who are most susceptible get infected early on. Whatever the reason, the studies dealt mostly with couples who'd been together for a while.

These studies most often look at what we might call "survivor" couples: couples who've, up until that point, not transmitted the herpes virus. It could be that there's something about the immune responses of the individuals involved that makes them less vulnerable to getting herpes in the first place—we just don't know. But it may not be accurate to apply their risks to the risks of couples who've been together for a shorter period of time.

LOWERING THE RISK OF TRANSMISSION

Are you ready for an analogy? Let's say you want to avoid being killed in a car accident, so you routinely do several things to keep that from happening: you wear a seat belt, you've taken drivers' education classes, you don't drink and drive, you don't drive when sleepy or when taking certain medications, and you observe traffic safety laws (well, most of the time). In short, you do a combination of things to protect yourself and your passengers.

When you're trying to prevent the transmission of genital herpes, you can take this same sort of multipronged approach. One large and well-respected research study (Corey et al. 2004) found that if you take 500 milligrams of Valtrex (valacyclovir hydrochloride) once a day, you reduce the risk of transmission of genital HSV 2 by almost 50 percent. That's the only drug that's been evaluated for this purpose, but if Valtrex isn't covered by your insurance or there's some other barrier to using it, there's reason to believe, based on studies of viral shedding while on medication, that the other antiviral medicines acyclovir and famciclovir might work that way, too (Wald et al. 2006b).

Other studies found that using male condoms most of the time also reduces transmission by about half (Wald et al. 2001). Condoms aren't perfect, because they cover the shaft of the penis but not the base, the pubic hair area, or the scrotum. Also, condoms can break, so be sure to use an adequate amount and the correct type of lubrication (not petroleum-based products), and use condoms that are fresh and not dried out by heat, the sun, or years in your wallet. Most condoms now have expiration dates, so check those carefully. Use latex or polyurethane condoms rather than animal skin when possible. Put the condom on right away, when there's a full erection; having a little genital-to-genital contact with an uncovered penis before intercourse offers an opportunity for transmission. Don't unroll the condom before you put it on; place the unrolled condom on the head of the penis with the unrolled portion on the outside. Leave a little room at the tip if there's none built in, and carefully unroll, trying not to leave air bubbles underneath. When ejaculation is over, hold the condom onto the bottom of the penis so that it doesn't slip off the now-softer penis before pulling out of the vagina or anus. Condoms are very helpful at reducing transmission of HSV but only if they're used correctly and consistently.

Learning to recognize outbreaks also reduces the risk of transmission, though we don't have statistics showing how useful this is. For example, if you believe that the crack you get on your labia every few months is a yeast infection, you won't feel the need to avoid sex when you have it. But if you learn that it really is herpes, you'll avoid sex during times when you have that crack in the skin. That's one less time when the active virus is present that you'll place your partner at risk.

Finally, we know that the simple act of telling your partner before you have sex that you have herpes reduces the risk of transmission. Dr. Anna Wald did an elegant but simple study on the benefits of knowing that your partner has herpes. She asked people with proven first-episode infection this simple question: "Did you or did you not know when you had sex with the person who infected you that he or she had genital herpes?" If the answer was "Yes, I knew," the average time from starting to have sex to acquiring herpes was about 240 days. If the answer was "No, I didn't know," the average time to acquisition was about 60 days (Wald et al. 2006a).

Do the benefits of daily suppressive therapy add to those of condom use? We can't be sure about that, but intuitively, it would seem so. If you take medicine to reduce the amount of virus present in the genitals and then you cover whatever virus is left with a condom, it seems to me that you've got what's called a "cumulative impact," though the research on this issue couldn't confirm this, due to low numbers of patients who took daily medicine and used condoms regularly (Corey et al. 2004). For example, if you start with a risk of transmission of about 10 percent per year from male to female, and you add daily antiviral therapy, you reduce the risk to about 5 percent per year (almost a 50 percent reduction). If you then add regular condom use, you reduce the risk again by about 50 percent, so you're down to about 2.5 percent. Beginning to recognize outbreaks and making sure your partner knows you have herpes likely provide even more benefit, though we can't say how much. Looking at this another way, if you do everything we've talked about and you started with a risk of about 10 percent per year, the chance of *not* transmitting is more than 90 to 95 percent in a year! That's really very good.

DISCUSSING TRANSMISSION WITH YOUR PARTNER

Now that you know what behaviors put you at risk of infecting others, as well as the levels of risk, you need to know what to do to reduce the risk. Here are some questions to discuss with your partner that might get at some underlying concerns about the transmission of herpes.

- On a scale of 1 to 10, how worried is each of us about transmission?

- What would be the worst thing about transmitting herpes?

- As a couple, what are we willing to do to avoid transmission?

- Are we willing to give up this relationship over the risk of transmitting herpes?

Questions for the Uninfected Partner

Here are five additional questions for the uninfected partner to think about, along with some "food for thought" I provided after each question:

If I decide not to take the risk of getting herpes and to leave this relationship, what are my chances of running into this problem again? Look back at the Herpes Simplex Virus Type 2 Seroprevalence 1999–2004 chart in chapter 2, which shows how many people in a specific age group and gender have herpes; which is the group you would most likely get involved with in a new relationship? Remember, too, that 90 percent of people with genital herpes in that group don't know they're infected. So if you decide to move on and find a partner who doesn't have herpes, it would be important that all your future potential sex partners be tested prior to sexual activity or you could find yourself in an even riskier situation. The person who knows he or she has herpes can do something about it, such as alert you to the issue, take daily medicine, suggest that condoms be used to reduce transmission, and avoid sex when herpes symptoms are present. But the person who's infected but doesn't know it won't do any of those things, so in that case, your risk of getting herpes will be much higher.

How do I thoughtfully balance the prospect of a loving life with my partner who has genital herpes against the risk of my contracting herpes, which I would have forever, even if we don't end up staying together? That's the $64,000 question, isn't it? And the answer will vary a great deal from one person to another. When I'm having trouble with a decision, I sometimes take a piece of paper and make columns for the pros and cons; in this case, one column could be headed "Pros of taking the risk and being with my partner," and the other could be "Cons of taking the risk of getting herpes." On the "pro" side, you could list the things you value about the relationship and about your partner, the relatively small statistical risk of getting herpes, the effective tools for reducing the risk of infection, management strategies if you did get infected, and so on. On the "con" side, you might note things like worrying about getting herpes when you make love, having to deal with outbreaks if you got infected, how having herpes would affect your view of yourself as a sexual being, and having to tell new partners about your herpes if you got infected and didn't stay together.

If I stay with my partner for the long term, will I be certain to get herpes eventually? No. In fact, some researchers believe that uninfected people in long-term relationships with partners who are infected develop an immune response that may actually offer them some protection against infection (Posavad et al. 2003). The risk of getting herpes probably doesn't accumulate over time; it begins and ends with each sexual encounter. The more sexual encounters one has, the greater the risk, but only because there are more opportunities, not because somehow these events accumulate.

What if I stay with my partner and I get herpes, and then we break up? Won't it be harder for me to find a new partner if I'm infected? Maybe. It's something to consider. At a minimum, you may feel some anxiety about telling future partners that you have herpes. Mostly, I don't hear that people are rejected because they have herpes, but every now and then someone declines to take the risk and moves on, and that isn't easy on the self-esteem. When counseling discordant couples, I've noticed that uninfected partners who have the most difficulty handling the risk of getting herpes tend to be individuals for whom sexuality is a big part of what defines them. This is probably a silly analogy, but it's kind of like a hand model who might be willing to engage in activities that put the legs or body at risk of injury but not the hands.

My partner gets frequent and painful outbreaks. If I get herpes from my partner, will my outbreaks be as severe? The current thinking on this question is that it's an individual's immune response that defines how severe the outbreaks are, not the particular virus itself. I've seen patients with no outbreaks at all who were infected by partners who had twelve outbreaks per year.

Over the years I've been asked many questions about the transmission of herpes. In fact, transmission is the second most common topic I'm asked about on WebMD (diagnosis is the first). Following are examples of a few of the more common questions.

COMMONLY ASKED QUESTIONS ABOUT HERPES TRANSMISSION

I have genital HSV 1, and my partner gets cold sores, which we assume is also HSV 1. If he has intercourse with me, can he get HSV 1 genitally? And will I get cold sores on my mouth if I kiss him? We believe it's very unlikely that either of you would get a new infection with the same type of virus at a different place on the body after your first infection is well established. I've not seen that happen in a patient, and unfortunately, blood tests can't help us answer that question. I wouldn't worry about getting HSV 1 in a new location on your body if you have it already.

My partner and I met on a herpes dating website. We both have HSV 2, and it's really nice not to have worry about having "the Talk," but I'm wondering if there's more than one strain of HSV 2, and should we be concerned about that? The last thing I need is more herpes! Yes, there is more than one strain of HSV 2, but this is probably not an issue, because once you have an immune response to HSV 2, it's highly unlikely that you'll get a new strain of the same virus. If a person does get more than one strain of the HSV 2 virus, it doesn't appear to cause more frequent or severe outbreaks. It seems that your own immune response is the most important factor in how your herpes virus behaves, not the virus itself.

This viral shedding business really has me down and confused. I'm in tune with my body. I know it well, and I can't believe that it could give off virus without my being aware of it. Are there some people, like me, who really don't have shedding without symptoms? No, we believe that virtually everyone who has HSV 2 infection sheds at certain times without knowing that it's happening. Do you think that if you had high blood pressure, you could feel that in your body? No, that's something that can only be determined by taking your blood pressure. Do you think that if you had breast cancer, you'd know right away? No. You get mammograms, because cancer can start before you could feel a lump or detect a nipple discharge. There are many other examples, but my point is that you can only know your body so well. Parts of it you can't know at all, no matter how vigilant and perceptive you are. Shedding is something that happens at the cellular level. You're a normal person with non-microscopic powers of perception. You can only do the best you can, and some things are simply outside your ability to perceive and control. You'll do better if you accept that fact and just cope with the impact of potential transmission as best you can with the tools we've discussed. Part of the frustration around this subject of shedding may really be your feeling of loss of control, and I completely understand and sympathize with that.

I have HSV 2 genitally and test negative for HSV 1, and my partner has tested negative for HSV 2 but has oral herpes. Can I give her my HSV 2 by kissing her? Will I get her HSV 1 by kissing her? No and no. Think about your body parts that are infected and where they'll be encountering your partner's. Your penis is infected, right? That genital virus won't come up through your body and out through your mouth to infect your partner. It'll stay in its own nerve group, and you'll be infectious only from the genital area. And it appears that having HSV 2 largely protects you against getting HSV 1 (Brown et al. 1997), so that's good news, right?

I get herpes outbreaks only on my buttocks. Can I safely cover the sores with a bandage and have sex with my partner without worrying about infecting him genitally? I've never had a genital outbreak, so I'm pretty sure I have buttocks herpes, not genital herpes. First, "buttocks herpes" *is* genital herpes. Remember that genital herpes comes into your body through a sexual contact and takes up residence in that group of nerves at the base of your spine. But when it makes travel plans to come to the skin again, it can come out on any branch of that nerve group. The buttocks area is in that nerve-group area, and when herpes is active, it's active. About 20 percent of the time that you're having a buttocks outbreak, you're also shedding virus from your genitals (Kerkering et al. 2006). Just because your outbreaks are only on the buttocks doesn't mean you can't infect someone else through sex. You can. Bandaging won't prevent transmission to your partner.

Hey, it's me again, from the question above. I don't like your answer very much, but I do get it. So here's another question about shedding. I love to spoon with my partner when sleeping—my butt snuggled against his front, if you get the picture. Do I have to worry about shedding virus from my bottom if I have no outbreak at the time? You'll like this answer better. No, when you're symptom free, you can still spoon without worrying about shedding. The thicker skin on your buttocks doesn't shed virus as does the thin skin of the penis, vagina, or labia. Shedding is not a concern from buttocks skin, thigh skin, or abdominal skin during times when you have no symptoms. If you spoon when you sleep, and the penis touches your genitals, it's not a big deal, but if it tends to happen a lot, you might want to wear pj's when you have outbreaks anyway.

I'm a sixty-year-old guy, my wife and I've been married for a long time, and I have HSV 2. We took your advice this year and finally got her tested, and she's negative for HSV 2. We're so happy together, and I'm glad she isn't infected. We've been really careful about not having sex if I have even a little twinge, and I use condoms almost every time we have sex. But to tell the truth, as I get older, condoms seem to work against my erections, if you get my drift. They really do interfere with my sexual pleasure and hers. I take antiviral medication like clockwork and get outbreaks very infrequently. She'd like to stop worrying about herpes—stop the condoms and stop examining my penis with a bright light every time we want to make love—but we're good with the daily medicine. I'm definitely willing to continue to protect her with our usual routine if that's the right thing to do, but I wonder if the benefits really outweigh the risks at this point in our lives together. Is this a bad decision on our part? Absolutely not! I imagine that the bright-light drill, in particular, gets pretty old over time. And lots of men have more trouble using condoms as they get older. There's no one right answer about the transmission question—and there's no rule that says herpes must be prevented at any cost. The sex police won't come knocking on your door if you choose to stop worrying about herpes. Let's be really clear about that. If couples decide they want to abandon the tools to reduce transmission, that's completely up to them. You've experienced that herpes can be well managed from a physical point of view, and she knows what's up and wants this change just as you do. So make it, and enjoy your sex lives even more. One problem with your question is that some women reading this will write to me and ask, "Where in the world do I find a great guy like him?" and I won't have the answer to that question. See what you started?

I hope this clarifies for you some of the issues involved in herpes transmission. It may take going back and rereading certain sections a few times to ingrain the information solidly in your head. It can be quite complicated to think about body parts connecting in various combinations, type 1 and type 2, what places are vulnerable, and how the virus is given off from them. You'll eventually get it though, and then you'll feel more in control of the transmission possibilities.

Chapter 4

Diagnosis: Certainty Is the Starting Point

You might think diagnosing genital herpes would be the easy part, but it turns out that a herpes diagnosis isn't always simple, and it isn't always done correctly. Various clinicians diagnose it quite differently, and accuracy of diagnosis varies widely. Before you can move ahead and adjust to having herpes, you need to know for sure that your diagnosis was accurate.

UNDERSTANDING HOW HERPES IS DIAGNOSED

Right now you might be asking yourself questions like these: Why is it up to *me* to sort this out? Why can't I just assume that my clinician's diagnosis was correct? Why are you going on and on about diagnosing herpes in a book for those of us who already have it? The answer to all of these questions is that things have changed rapidly over the years regarding herpes diagnosis, and not all clinicians use the most modern and reliable tests. Some don't even use lab tests and rely instead on a visual examination to make their diagnoses. Much of the time, they're correct, but a visual diagnosis has limitations, depends greatly on the clinician's skill, and, when used alone without lab tests, is wrong about 20 percent of the time (Langenberg et al. 1999). That's why, beginning in 2002, the Centers for Disease Control and Prevention (CDC) (2006) recommended that every herpes diagnosis be supported by a lab test, not just a visual examination, and that the test be type specific; that is, one that can distinguish HSV 1 from 2. If you were diagnosed ten years ago or more, tests were much less accurate then, and many tests used today weren't even available that long ago.

Since your body and your future are in the balance, it's in your best interest to be certain you received a correct diagnosis. It's even possible that you're reading this book to help you deal with herpes, but will later find out (from the steps you'll be prompted to take in this chapter) that you don't have herpes at all. It's also possible that you've been told you have HSV 2 based on the location of your symptoms, and you really have HSV 1. So we'll talk about how diagnosis should be done and how to know if yours was correct.

In addition to being certain about your own diagnosis, I'm telling you about diagnostic tests, because you may be in situations with partners in which you'll need to know these things. You might meet people who say they don't have herpes but have never actually been tested. After reading what follows, you'll know which tests would be useful for them. You might meet people who know they have genital herpes but have never learned what type of virus they have. To determine your risk of infecting each other, a lab test that includes typing is necessary, so it's important to know which test is best.

There are three ways clinicians diagnose herpes: a visual diagnosis (with or without a lab test), virus swab tests, and blood antibody tests. All three methods are greatly enhanced by the inclusion of a frank and factual sexual history, and a thorough physical examination.

Physical Examination

I've often heard from clinicians: "Herpes is clearly herpes; I don't need a lab test to confirm the obvious." It turns out, however, that the old idea about "typical herpes" wasn't all that accurate. For years we believed that genital herpes was always obvious, that everyone with a first infection knew exactly when it happened; that he or she had multiple, painful genital lesions that were always caused by HSV 2; and that anyone without these "typical herpes symptoms" didn't really have it. It turns out, of course, that genital herpes has many different appearances—some dramatic, but most quite subtle and often not caused by HSV 2. If clinicians rely only on what they see with their eyes, sometimes they are mistaken. Did someone just look at your genitals and tell you that you had herpes? If so, I strongly recommend getting a lab test to confirm the opinion.

Did your clinician gather a detailed history of all symptoms you've had and the sexual activities you participated in over the last three to four months prior to your visit? These should've been very personal questions about what body parts of yours came in contact with what body parts of others, how long ago, and how often. Were condoms used or any other barrier method? Did your partner report any history of genital herpes then or since? Because herpes can be transmitted through oral sex, vaginal intercourse, anal sex, or simply by genital-to-genital rubbing, you should've been asked about all these possibilities.

A complete exam for a woman should include an inspection of the cervix and vagina with a speculum, as well as an exam of the external genitals, pubic area, and anus. If painful lesions are present, an internal exam with a speculum might be too painful, so that's often postponed until the tenderness diminishes. That's okay, because it isn't absolutely necessary to see inside. For men, the entire penis, scrotum, anus, and pubic-hair area are typically examined for signs of problems. And this applies whether they have sex with men or women. A good exam also inspects the thighs, buttocks, groin, lymph nodes, and mouth of both men and women.

If no lesions are present, the exam alone can't rule out herpes. In other words, a person could have genital herpes, but since herpes isn't symptomatic all the time, a clinician could easily miss it when relying solely on an exam.

Even if symptoms are present, the visual exam is only the beginning of a diagnosis. Clinicians make errors. It happens all the time, and although your clinician may have wonderful diagnostic skills, mistakes can happen. A lab test is essential for the diagnosis of genital herpes, even if symptoms are present that look like herpes. And finally, an exam can't distinguish HSV 1 from 2. Some clinicians have the mistaken belief that everything below the waist is HSV 2, but now we know that many new genital herpes cases are caused by HSV 1. Since you've probably already been diagnosed with herpes, at the end of this chapter is a list of questions to ask your clinician if you have any doubts about the accuracy of your diagnosis.

But which lab tests can provide an accurate diagnosis? I'm so glad you asked!

Virus Swab Tests

If you have symptoms present at the time of the exam, a swab test should be gathered from the area showing symptoms. Swab tests are gathered only when a person is showing symptoms; this is not a screening test that can be done anytime. Only a swab test can confirm *where* someone is infected, not just *if* that person is infected. The blood tests we discuss later can tell you whether you're infected but can't always tell you where. But which swab test is best? Here are the available options and a discussion of their accuracy. But before we go there, let's define some terms:

False negative: The person really is infected with herpes, but the test result shows negative.

False positive: The person really isn't infected with herpes, but the test shows positive.

True positive: The person is infected with herpes, just as the test shows.

True negative: The person isn't infected with herpes, just as the test shows.

Sensitivity of the test: If a test is 98 percent sensitive, it means that out of 100 people who have herpes, the test will identify 98 of them but miss 2.

Specificity of the test: This is a difficult concept to grasp; it has to do with a test's ability to identify people who are truly negative for some condition. Take, for example, the specificity of the herpes antibody test: out of 100 people who actually don't have herpes, 97 will have a negative test, but 3 will have a positive test. This means the test has 97 percent specificity.

Viral Culture

For many years, we relied on a swab test called *viral culture* to diagnose herpes. A culture is gathered with a swab that's rubbed aggressively over a visible sore or break in the skin. I know—you're crossing your legs and thinking, "Ouch!" But gentle swabbing just doesn't give as accurate a result as does swabbing "with gusto." It's necessary to rub firmly to recover enough cells to get a good sample. But short-term pain brings long-term gain, if the result is a more accurate lab test, right?

For a viral culture, the specimen is gathered and sent to the laboratory, where healthy animal cells are combined with the patient's sample. A laboratory technician observes the culture for specific changes that typically appear when herpes is present. If the classic changes *do* occur, the test is declared positive, meaning that herpes simplex virus is present in the sample. Typing should then be done on every positive sample to see if the patient has HSV 1 or 2. Remember, about 40 percent of new genital herpes cases are type 1, not type 2 (Gupta, Warren, and Wald 2007). False-positive cultures (the culture says herpes is present, but it really isn't present) are extremely rare. If a culture test gathered from lesions comes back with positive results, the person can be clear that he or she really does have herpes.

If the changes in the animal cells at the lab don't occur within a certain period, usually three to fourteen days, the sample is declared negative. This means one of two things: either no virus was present in the sample to make the test turn positive, or there wasn't sufficient virus to make the test turn positive. This doesn't necessarily mean, however, that the person doesn't have herpes. There are several reasons why a viral culture might be falsely negative (the person is infected, but the culture result is negative):

- The culture sample could've been gathered too late in the outbreak so that the sores were too healed to yield active virus.

- The clinician who gathered the swab wasn't aggressive enough in swabbing to gather an adequate sample.

- The culture may have been handled inappropriately in the medical office or lab, or it may have taken too long for the sample to arrive at the lab after it was collected.

- The number of virus particles present in the sample wasn't sufficient to make the culture turn positive.

One study at the University of Washington found a 76 percent false-negative rate for cultures when compared to the better test, PCR (polymerase chain reaction), which we'll discuss next (Wald et al. 2003). That means that, about three out of four times that a culture came back negative, the person really *did* have herpes but the culture failed to pick it up. All negative swab results, whether culture or PCR, from people suspected of having genital herpes should be followed up with an accurate type-specific blood test (which we'll discuss soon) three to four months from possible infection to see if the person really does have herpes.

PCR (Polymerase Chain Reaction)

PCR swab testing is performed just like a culture: a specimen is gathered with a swab from an abnormal area of skin. Usually, the same collection materials are used that are used for a culture. However, PCR is far more sensitive than culture, meaning that more cases of herpes are picked up by PCR than by culture. PCR takes a tiny piece of virus and amplifies, or copies, it many times so that it can be identified and subsequently typed as HSV 1 or 2. For now, PCR is available in fewer labs than culture, and is typically more expensive, but it's much more likely than the culture test to pick up infection. The two largest labs in the United States (Quest Diagnostics and LabCorp) do herpes PCR testing, so that's a good sign of things to come. Transport issues don't influence PCR results as they do culture results, so variations in temperature or the length of travel time to the lab won't affect PCR results as they do culture results.

One problem with the PCR test is that there's not yet an FDA-approved standardized version of the test, and some insurance companies may not cover non-FDA-approved tests. However, we haven't experienced this as a problem for reimbursement in our clinic at all.

Culture vs. PCR

In the future, culture will likely be replaced completely by PCR, as happened several years ago with gonorrhea and chlamydia testing. Only PCR should be used to test spinal fluid or to diagnose babies with suspected herpes infections. Are you wondering if your swab test was PCR or culture? Look at the paper copy of your test results; if it says, "HSV isolated," it's a culture test. If it says, "HSV DNA detected," it's a PCR test. If your swab-test results were positive, regardless of the method used, you should believe them. If your swab test was negative, remember that neither culture nor PCR is perfect. You may need to have an antibody test to sort things out; we'll talk more about that later in this chapter.

Tzanck Smear

The Tzanck smear is sometimes used in public STI clinics for a quick diagnosis, or it may be used for a preliminary in-house diagnosis in dermatology offices while the culture or PCR is being run at the lab. For this test, cells from a lesion are collected on a swab, placed on a glass slide, stained, and examined under a microscope. Cells infected with herpes virus appear very large with many centers (also known as *multinucleated giant cells*), and infected cells pick up the stain in a different way than uninfected ones do. This test isn't as desirable as culture or PCR, but a positive Tzanck read by an experienced lab, combined with an accurate health and sexual history, physical exam, and the presence of lesions, could be considered reasonably accurate.

A negative Tzanck smear is not definitive. Tzanck smears pick up about 60 percent of the actual herpes cases, as compared to PCR swabs (Nahass et al. 1992). And Tzanck smears can't be typed: they won't tell you if you have HSV 1 or 2, and they can also confuse HSV 1 or 2 with varicella-zoster infection, because the stained cells look the same. As with the other swab tests, if a negative result is obtained, it should be followed three to four months after possible infection with an accurate type-specific blood test to determine if herpes infection has actually occurred.

Pap Smear

Some women reading this book have been told they have herpes based on a Pap smear. Pap smears use a staining process similar to the Tzanck test, but a slightly different technique is used and cells are gathered from the cervix, not from a sore. Pap smears look for cervical cancer, but sometimes other infections can be seen on the same slide. A herpes diagnosis from a Pap smear usually goes something like this: no herpes symptoms are noted at the time of the yearly exam, but when the Pap smear results come back, the pathologist who reads the slide notes something like, "Cells suggestive of herpes simplex are noted on the Pap smear." This notation should trigger further herpes testing (like antibody testing or swab testing) from any sore that might show up later. A herpes diagnosis from a Pap smear should not stand alone.

Silver Pap

A few labs are starting to use a new test that bundles herpes PCR testing with a Pap smear and testing for gonorrhea, chlamydia, and perhaps other diseases as well. Its sometimes called a *silver Pap*. It's important to understand what's going on here, and trust me, it isn't good. The herpes PCR part of the Pap test looks to see if HSV is present at the time the Pap smear is gathered. If the test is positive, then, yes, the woman has herpes. But if the test is negative for herpes, that doesn't mean she doesn't have it; it simply means there was no herpes virus present on the cervix at the time the sample was gathered. It's a little like my seeing a woman working at her desk, and saying, "That woman's not a chess player." My thinking was, "Hey, she's not playing chess right now, so she must not be a chess player." Of course, that doesn't make any sense. People are more likely to play chess at home or on break. Just because they aren't playing chess when I see them at work doesn't say a thing about their chess playing; it just says that *at that moment*, they aren't chess players, not that they never are. Unlike gonorrhea or chlamydia, herpes virus isn't present all the time on the cervix, so a negative silver Pap with herpes PCR testing included really doesn't tell us anything for certain. The only way to know about herpes infection when there are no symptoms at the time of the test is to look for antibody to the virus, not the virus itself. Remember that when a person is infected with herpes, the virus is only present on the genital skin or mucous membrane from time to time, not *all* the time. Antibody, on the other hand, can consistently be found in the blood, whether a person does or doesn't have symptoms. Avoid herpes testing from a Pap smear. You could be falsely reassured.

Blood Antibody Tests

The exciting thing in herpes diagnosis right now is type-specific blood tests that look for herpes antibody. *Antibody* is a protein your body makes in response to being infected with a virus. Despite what anyone else may tell you, there's no such thing as a blood test's being positive due to mere exposure to a virus. Let's use the analogy of a positive pregnancy test. A pregnancy test isn't positive because a woman has been exposed to semen (obviously, she has); it's positive because she's pregnant, and a positive herpes antibody test is the same: it means you're both infected and infectious to others.

It can take a while for the body to make herpes antibody, so it's important to wait long enough after possible infection to draw the blood sample for greatest accuracy. The ideal wait is four months after possible infection. I used to ask patients who came for herpes screening, "When was the last time you had a possible exposure to herpes?" They'd say, "Oh, maybe a year ago." So I'd ask, "So you haven't had sex in a year?" And they'd answer, "No, I had sex last week but not with anyone who'd have genital herpes!" Now, instead, I ask, "When was the last time you had any kind of sexual contact?" That's important for determining the right timing for their herpes antibody tests. People with herpes don't wear little tags that read, "I'm infected." As previously mentioned, almost 90 percent of people who have HSV 2 don't even know they have it, so deciding who has or doesn't have herpes based on what they tell you, how they look, how much education they have, or how much money they make just doesn't cut it. Only a blood antibody test can tell who has herpes and who doesn't.

Outdated and Potentially Inaccurate Blood Tests

The outdated, old-style blood antibody tests (known as *crude antigen* tests) can detect antibody to herpes simplex in general but are poor at distinguishing type 1 from type 2. So if a person has either cold-sore virus or genital herpes, the blood test is positive for herpes antibody—period. These outdated tests are particularly misleading, because they seem to *imply* that they can tell the difference between HSV 1 and 2, but they really can't. You have to read the fine print to find that out. So people could be told they have HSV 2 (almost always genital herpes) when they really have HSV 1 (still most often a cold-sore virus, yet it could be genital). This inability to distinguish between the two viruses is called *cross-reactivity*, which is why these tests should never be used. You would think that with the availability of the newer tests, these old ones would be off the market, but they're still used in some labs, so you'll have to do your homework to determine which test was done for you.

IgM (a different kind of antibody—with an *M* this time) blood tests don't accurately distinguish between the types of herpes virus and can't accurately tell a new infection from an old one. Unfortunately, many clinicians still order them. In fact, it's probably the biggest mistake clinicians make when doing herpes testing. IgM tests for herpes simplex may also mistakenly pick up other herpes viruses like chicken pox or mono. IgM tests for herpes diagnosis in adults should be avoided completely.

Type-Specific Serologic Tests

The new tests, called *type-specific serologic tests* (or *TSSTs*), *do* distinguish between HSV 1 and 2 with a high degree of certainty, by detecting antibodies to a protein that differs between HSV 1 and 2. This protein is *glycoprotein G* (or *gG*), and the tests are sometimes referred to as the *glycoprotein G specific*, or *gG-based*, *tests*. These new, highly accurate tests all measure a kind of antibody called IgG (lots of *G*'s, huh?) and don't falsely detect antibody from other herpes viruses, like chicken pox. So clinicians who say they don't do blood tests because the tests can't sort out genital herpes from chicken pox aren't familiar with the newest blood antibody tests for herpes simplex virus. You might want to show them this chapter to bring them up to speed.

Western blot: The *Western blot* herpes antibody test was developed at the University of Washington (UW) by Rhoda Ashley-Morrow. In the United States, this test is still only available through the University of Washington, but you don't have to go to Seattle to get it done. Your blood sample can be sent through larger national labs like Quest Diagnostics or LabCorp, which have offices throughout the country, or it can be sent directly from your clinician's office to the UW. The Western blot test looks at the individual proteins that make up the antibody to herpes, so it's quite technical and complex compared to other tests. It isn't an automated test; three separate technicians read the test to reach a result. The UW website, which is listed in chapter 11, tells how your clinician can send a sample to the lab. You might want this test if:

- Your other test results aren't completely clear or your HerpeSelect antibody test (discussed in the next section) has a low positive value (1.1 to 3.5), and you want confirmation of the result.

- You don't believe you really have herpes, and you need a "second opinion" in the form of a lab test. It's okay to get another test done if it helps you believe the original diagnosis.

- You had a positive swab test for herpes that wasn't typed, but your antibody test came back negative for HSV 1 and 2. What's going on here? The Western blot test is slightly more sensitive than the HerpeSelect tests for HSV 1 and will sometimes catch HSV 1 antibody that the HerpeSelect tests miss.

- You read somewhere (like in this book) that the Western blot is the "gold standard" test. This type-specific test was around long before the others, and because the analysis is more complex than others, the Western blot can be valuable if any part of the diagnosis is confusing to you or your clinician.

HerpeSelect: HerpeSelect is a brand name, not a kind of test, but because it was the only type-specific test around for a long time, you might sometimes see it used as a test name. The HerpeSelect blood antibody tests (there are separate tests for HSV 1 and 2) can accurately distinguish between HSV 1 and 2, and they're very good at picking up herpes antibody. There are actually three tests that fall into the HerpeSelect brand: ELISA, Immunoblot, and Express.

The HerpeSelect *ELISA* tests for HSV 1 and 2 provide a number result called an *index value*. This table shows the index values associated with a negative, an equivocal, and a positive result.

<0.9	Negative
0.9–1.1	Equivocal
>1.1	Positive

When you get a negative result, there's almost never a 0 value because of the way the test is run, so don't panic if there's some numeric value associated with a negative result. What really matters is if the value falls below 0.9 or rises above 1.1. My clinic runs twenty-five or so ELISA tests each week, and I can count on one hand the number of 0 values we've seen in our lab. It has nothing to do with being infected "a little" (which you now know is impossible); if it's less than 0.9, your test is negative.

If your number falls between 0.9 and 1.1, the result is called *equivocal*, which just means that the result is unclear and another ELISA test, or a different confirmatory test, should be run later. If you have the ELISA test done again and the number goes down, the result is negative. If it goes up, the result could be positive. Rarely does a second test fall into the equivocal area. If it does and at least four months have gone by since the time of possible infection, you might want to consider a Western blot test for confirmation, but your test result is likely negative.

An index value above 1.1 is considered positive. However, research has found that sometimes when a person has an index value that falls between 1.1 and 3.5 (low positive), it could be a false positive (the test says you have herpes, but you really don't) (Golden et al. 2005). If you have a low positive value on your ELISA test, I recommend that you get a different kind of test, preferably the Western blot. If you've been told you have herpes based on a blood antibody test alone, with no positive swab test and no symptoms of genital herpes, and you've had little risk of infection, I strongly suggest that you get a copy of the lab test results to see if it was a HerpeSelect ELISA. If the value was below 3.5, I hope you'll get another test to confirm the positive result.

The second style of HerpeSelect test is the *Immunoblot*. Immunoblot results have no number associated with them, just a positive or negative result. This style of test might be run in a smaller laboratory that runs few herpes antibody tests. Positive and negative results are decided based on a color change on a strip of paper that indicates the presence or absence of antibody to HSV 1, 2, or both.

The third test in the HerpeSelect family is the *Express*. It was designed for use during a visit to a clinician's office. It takes about fifteen minutes to run and looks for HSV 2 antibody only, not HSV 1, so if you need to know about both types, this isn't the test for you. If you've had a history of recurrent cold sores on your lip, chin, or nose, you already know you have HSV 1 and don't need an antibody test to tell you that. But don't confuse canker sores with cold sores. Canker sores occur inside your mouth, often near the gum line, and you might associate their occurrence with eating certain foods. Canker sores are not caused by herpes.

Biokit: The *Biokit* test is also done in the clinician's office and takes about five minutes, with accuracy close to that of the HerpeSelect tests. Like the HerpeSelect Express, it also looks only for HSV 2.

Captia: The Trinity Biotech company makes a test called *Captia*. The test performance is similar to the others. It's been in regular use since 2007, so compared to the other tests, it's a relative newcomer.

Timing Is Everything

With all herpes blood antibody tests, timing is everything. Because the blood tests look for antibody, which is something your body makes and not something you get from someone else, enough time must pass between infection and testing for enough antibodies to be made and detected by the tests. Pregnancy testing is similar. If you do a pregnancy test too soon after conception, it may be negative. If done two weeks later, the result may be positive. In the same way, herpes antibody tests must be done after enough time has passed. This table (Ashley-Morrow, Krantz, and Wald 2003) shows how accurate testing for herpes is in relationship to when the infection occurred.

3 weeks after infection	50% of those infected will test positive.
6 weeks after infection	70% of those infected will test positive.
16 weeks after infection	Almost everyone who is infected will test positive.

Obviously, if you test too soon after possible infection and the test result comes up negative, you'll believe incorrectly that you don't have herpes. Sometimes, however, testing right after a worrisome sexual encounter can give you some useful "baseline" information, like what was going on with you before the encounter. For example, Susan has a new sex partner, but she doesn't get tested before they have sex. She then waits four months to get tested and is positive for HSV 2. Was Susan infected prior to having sex with her new partner, or did her new partner infect her with HSV 2? In this situation, there's really no way to know. But if Susan had had a negative herpes antibody test before having sex with her new partner, or within a few days afterward, and four months later was tested again with a positive result for HSV 2, she'd know that she was newly infected and who had infected her, assuming she'd had no sexual contact with anyone else around the same time.

Identifying New vs. Old Infection

One common question people diagnosed with herpes have is: "How long have I had herpes?" A type-specific IgG blood test may help sort out a new from an old infection. Let's say someone develops a lesion in the genital area. A swab is gathered, and the swab test is positive for HSV 2. During the same visit, a blood sample is drawn, and the type-specific IgG antibody test comes back negative for HSV 2. This seeming "conflict" indicates that this is likely a first infection: there's virus present in the lesion, but not enough time has passed for antibody to the virus to be made. So that's a typical first infection: a positive swab test and a negative blood test for the same type. This combination of tests isn't always done, so don't be too disappointed if you look at your old results and don't find these two tests done on the same day. However, let's change the scene from above just a little bit. Let's say you develop a sore, and two weeks later you get a swab test and a blood antibody test done. The swab test and blood test are both positive. Because two weeks have passed, and antibody can be made that quickly, you can't know if you've been infected for a while or you just got a new infection.

What Type of Blood Test Did I Have?

Check out the actual lab paperwork if you've been diagnosed with herpes by a blood test. Get a copy of your test results to hold in your hand and look at. If you had an IgM test done, and it was positive but your IgG test was negative or not done, get retested with an IgG test now if it's been at least four months since the time of your original blood work. Your IgM test result may be a false positive. If your HerpeSelect ELISA result fell between 1.1 and 3.5, and you've had no symptoms associated with herpes and no positive swab test, get a second kind of confirmatory antibody test done, just to be sure.

Do I Need Blood Antibody Testing?

Who should have a blood antibody test for herpes? This is still somewhat controversial, but here's a partial list of situations that warrant one:

- If you had sex with someone who has herpes and want to know if you got infected, or you've met someone who has told you he or she has herpes and you want to know if you're at risk of getting infected.

- If you've been told from a visual exam alone that you have herpes and want to know if you really do. And remember that no one can tell HSV 1 from 2 just by looking. The lesions from both HSV 1 and 2 look identical, and both can be present "below the waist." For typing of the virus, you absolutely need a lab test.

- If you've had recurrent genital sores or similar symptoms but swab tests taken from the sores always come back negative for herpes. Remember, even the best swab tests (PCR) can give false negative results, especially with recurrent disease.

- If you've had repeated urinary-tract infection symptoms but your urine never grows any bacteria when it's sent to the lab for a culture. Several things could be going on here, but one is that you have herpes sores in the urethra, which causes pain during urination, because herpes lesions are open ulcers and urine is acidic, and—well, you get the picture. Ouch! In addition, there may be some pus (or white-blood) cells in the urine test, because herpes lesions have pus cells in them, and when urine passes over them, it picks up the pus cells and that gets detected in the urine test.

- If you want to get screened for *all* STIs, you should have a test for herpes too. You'll need to ask if herpes is included in the tests you'll have done, because even though herpes is the most prevalent STI in the United States today, many STI screens still don't include tests for herpes. Surprising, huh? Don't *assume* that your STI screen includes herpes testing—ask. The same is true for your "complete" physical exam or your pregnancy testing. Most don't look for herpes.

- If you're pregnant, it's important to know whether you have herpes and, if so, which type. We'll talk at length about the details in chapter 5.

- If you have HIV, you need to know if you have herpes too. If you're infected with both HSV 2 and HIV, your HIV infection can progress faster and make you even more likely to infect others with HIV. We'll talk in chapter 10 about other STIs and how all of that works.

QUESTIONS TO ASK YOUR CLINICIAN

As you read over the information about diagnosis, it's pretty normal to have questions about your own experience of getting diagnosed. It's really okay to ask your clinician additional questions, even if you don't get the feeling that these inquiries will be warmly received. It may be best to set up an appointment to go over lab results that are in your chart; it can take some time, and phone calls can feel rushed. I've included lists of questions that you might want to use when you talk to your clinician, one for if you've recently been diagnosed and your lab tests are still pending, and another for if you were diagnosed a while ago. Look these over and see which fits you.

Questions to Ask Your Clinician About Swab Tests

- Which test do you use for swabbing suspect skin lesions for herpes: culture or PCR (polymerase chain reaction)?

- Do you have the ability to use PCR tests instead of a culture test?

- Will you request typing of the virus (type 1 or type 2), or does that come automatically with each swab test?

- How long will it take to get the results back?

- Will you call me with the results, or should I call you?

Questions to Ask Your Clinician About Blood Antibody Testing

- Was the blood test you ordered an IgG test, an IgM test, or both? (If IgM testing was ordered, you may wish to ask that the test be canceled.)

- Was the IgG test type specific? Which specific test was ordered?

- How long will it take to get the results back on my test?

- Will you call me, or should I call you for the test results?

- Do you ever order confirmation on low-positive test results? Note: If your test result is low positive (1.1 to 3.5 index value on HerpeSelect) and you've never had any herpes symptoms, you could ask if confirmation can be ordered on this sample or another sample of your blood.

- Can I get a copy of my test results? How do I arrange that?

Questions to Ask Your Clinician About Your Past Herpes Diagnosis

- How was I diagnosed with genital herpes? Was it a swab test or a blood antibody test, or did I just have symptoms that looked like herpes?

- If I was diagnosed by a positive swab test, was typing performed on the sample (that is, was it determined to be herpes type 1 or 2)?

- If I was diagnosed by a blood antibody test, was it an IgG or an IgM blood antibody test?

- If the IgM was positive, was IgG testing done also? If yes, was it positive or negative?

- If the IgG test was also positive, was type 1 separate from type 2 on the results?

- If the HSV 2 test was positive, was there a numeric value to the result? If yes, what was the number?

Don't be too surprised if your clinician doesn't have all of these answers readily available. Herpes is of great interest to you personally, and you're doing lots of good reading to make sure you understand what's going on with your body. But your clinician may need a little time to come up with all the answers to these questions. And if you feel some resistance or defensiveness from your clinician, take a deep breath and politely and persistently keep asking your questions.

QUESTIONS AND ANSWERS ABOUT DIAGNOSING HERPES

People have more questions about diagnosis than any other aspect of genital herpes. Here are some typical questions I get on this topic:

I once had a severe rash in the genital area. A nurse practitioner took a look, told me it was herpes, and, because it was below my waist, said, "It's herpes type 2." I've only ever had sex with my husband, and he's only ever had it with me in our whole lives. I haven't had a recurrence of any symptoms in an entire year. What's up with that? I see why you're confused. First, the rash could've been many things, and if it's true that you and your husband have never had any sexual encounters with anyone else, HSV 2 is impossible. You could have genital HSV 1 infection if your husband gives you oral sex and is infected with oral herpes, but without a type-specific antibody test, you can't know for sure if you're infected with HSV 1. Even if you get a herpes antibody test now, it's positive for type 1, and you've never had a cold sore in your life, the HSV 1 antibody could've come from either an oral or a genital infection. The test won't tell where you're infected, only that you're infected. If your antibody test is positive for HSV 2, that can only mean that there have been other sexual partners for one or both of you, because HSV 2 is a sexually transmitted disease. If your blood antibody test is negative for both HSV 1 and 2, the rash you had was probably not herpes at all but something else altogether.

I had sores in the genital area about a year ago, and my doctor did a PCR swab test of them. The test was positive for herpes, but no typing was requested. I wanted to know about my type, because I'm planning on having sex with someone who has HSV 2. I had a blood antibody test drawn, but the antibody test was positive for HSV 1 only, and negative for HSV 2. Does this mean I have HSV 1 genitally? Yes, that's how you should interpret this result. You had virus present in the sore, so the swab test was positive, meaning that you have genital herpes. And since a lot of time has passed since your initial outbreak and the only antibody you have is HSV 1, the infection you have is genital HSV 1.

This next question is similar to the previous one:

My swab test from several sores was positive for herpes but wasn't typed. I was curious about the type because I've never had another sore, so I had a HerpeSelect antibody test a year later. It was completely negative for type 1 and type 2. Was my swab test wrong? I'm quite sure you do have genital herpes, but it may be genital HSV 1. The reason your antibody blood test came out negative is that the HerpeSelect test is only 91 percent sensitive for HSV 1 (from the product insert; see also www.ashastd.org/). That means that out of 100 actual cases of HSV 1 infection, the test only picks up 91 of them and misses almost 1 out of every 10, which is quite a lot. The HSV 2 test misses about 2 out of 100 cases, which is considerably better. My guess is that you fall into the 9 percent that the antibody test misses for HSV 1 infection. If you ever have another lesion, you may want to have it swabbed right away, and be sure it's typed this time. But for now, I believe you probably have HSV 1 genital herpes, but you can't really be sure from the HerpeSelect test what's going on here.

I've been married for twenty-five years, and last month I developed a group of blisters on my buttocks. The swab test taken from the blisters showed I have HSV 2 infection. I've never had anything like this before, only recurrent yeast infections. The blood test for antibody done on the same day was strongly positive. My husband got tested, and he's negative for HSV 2. Now he thinks I've been cheating on him, but I really haven't. I haven't had sex with anybody else for twenty-five years! I had other partners before we met but not since. He just doesn't believe me! It's not only possible but also fairly common to have had herpes for years without knowing it. It's also fairly common not to infect your partner, even after twenty-five years. My guess is that you got infected by an earlier partner and just never knew it. My second guess is that your recurrent yeast infections may have been herpes outbreaks. If your husband is open to doing a bit more reading, I think you'll be able to sort out the issues that herpes has raised in your marriage.

I was diagnosed by visual exam about three months ago. It was a pretty bad first infection: lots of sores, difficulty urinating, sensitivity to light, bad head-aches—the whole thing. After the first-episode treatment period of ten days, my doctor immediately put me on 1 gram of Valtrex a day so I wouldn't have any more bad outbreaks. Last week I went for an antibody test to be certain I have herpes and to try to figure out the type, and the antibody test was still completely negative. Was the diagnosis wrong? It's difficult to say. However, I recommend that you come off daily therapy and retest in a couple of months. Though the medication is helping you to avoid further outbreaks (if you really do have herpes), it's also possible that it could be interfering with the development of antibody by decreasing the rate of virus replication. If the virus isn't active very often because of the medicine, your immune system doesn't see it all that often, so it may take a little longer for your body to produce antibody. Try coming off the medicine, and test again in a few months.

I've never had any symptoms of genital herpes in my life, but I requested a full STI screen, because I'm going to start having sex with someone new. My last sexual encounter with someone else was three weeks ago. My HerpeSelect ELISA antibody test for HSV 2 came back with a value of 2.1. Is that a true positive result? Good question. Research shows that an ELISA value between 1.1 and 3.5 may be a false-positive result, and it should be con-firmed with a second test (Golden et al. 2005). You could have a low positive value because you've been recently infected (your latest encoun-ter being three weeks ago). I recommend not getting a second test right away but waiting about two months to get retested with the same ELISA type test. If your value is higher next time, you were likely *seroconverting* at the time of your first test, meaning that you were in the process of becoming antibody positive due to new infection. If, on the other hand, your test is still around 2.0, get a different kind of test, like the Western blot, to clarify your low positive value.

I have sores on my penis at least once a month, and they last two weeks. I know they're herpes, but all of my antibody tests and swab tests are negative for HSV 1 and 2. I paid for sex once, almost a year ago, and have had these symptoms ever since, and I just know they're herpes. Sometimes you have to look pretty closely to see them and use a very bright light, and it's easier to see them when I have an erection, but they're definitely there. Why won't the tests show that I have herpes? I've been to five doctors trying to get a positive diagnosis. Your tests are negative, because you almost certainly don't have herpes. You had an experience that was worrisome for you and may have created a sense of guilt and anxiety. You've been worried enough to seek five different opinions, and that's a lot. Start believing the test results. If you're really having sores, maybe a dermatologist can help you sort out the symptoms. And if the dermatologist tells you that you have normal penile skin, you should accept that. Sometimes, in a situation like yours, a person begins to notice a lot of skin features and sensations that were always there but now take on a "meaning." I'm not saying your symptoms are all in your head. I'm saying that they may be perfectly normal skin occurrences like hair follicles, pearly papules, plugged-up skin pores, or something else that's not herpes. Believing that you don't have herpes is a challenge, because you've convinced yourself that you're infected. Some professional help might even be needed to change your thinking about this. And, by the way, your situation is really quite common, and you aren't crazy. This will pass with time and maybe some counseling.

I got screened for all STIs, and my HSV 1 blood antibody test was positive, but my HSV 2 blood antibody test was negative. It's been six months since I've had any kind of sex at all. I've never had a cold sore in my life, but my ex-boyfriend, who gave me oral sex, had cold sores. I've never had any oral or genital symptoms at all. Do I have HSV 1 orally or genitally? The antibody test can only tell you whether or not you're infected, not where you're infected. We generally presume that HSV 2 infection is genital, because people who test positive for HSV 2 antibody shed virus from the genital tract quite often, even if they have no perceivable outbreaks. But HSV 1 is another matter—it can be oral or genital. Since you've never had a cold sore and have received oral sex from someone who did have cold sores, your infection could be either oral or genital. If you develop symptoms in either location, see your clinician right away for a swab test. Or ask if you can keep a swab-test kit at home, so you can gather a sample yourself at the first sign of an outbreak. Then you may find out if your infection is oral or genital. There's really no other way to know.

I tested positive for HSV 2 by antibody test at a value of greater than 5, but I've never had any herpes symptoms. My doctor says I've just been "exposed," but I think I'm really infected. Which is it, exposed or infected? And what does that mean in terms of future partners? Since your HSV 2 antibody test is firmly positive, you're infected. Obviously, you've also been exposed, which means that you're both infected and infectious to others. Now that you know you're infected with HSV 2, you may actually start to recognize symptoms you missed before. But even if you don't, consider yourself infectious to others.

I've had the ELISA blood test done three times now. My risky contact was six months ago. But I keep getting tested, because the HSV 2 values, though negative, seem to be moving upward, like .02, .08, .17. I'm not taking any medicine or anything, but this trend upward worries me. What does this mean? The negative numbers don't mean anything by themselves. The numbers are supposed to vary, because they come about as a comparison to a control that's present in the test kit. They aren't going upward, they're all negative, and you need to stop testing now. You don't have HSV 2.

I'm seventy-two years old. I've had a group of painful, itchy blisters show up on my buttocks every few months for years now. They last about ten days, get a crust, and go away. My doctor says they're recurrent shingles, and I know that shingles is herpes, right? I'm wondering if I should get the shingles vaccine to help me cope with them every few months. Would that help? Let's back up just a minute. Shingles (or varicella-zoster) is a reactivation of the chicken pox virus. Only 3 percent of people who get shingles once ever get it again, and almost none get it a third time (Gnann Jr. and Whitley 2002). So what you have is almost certainly not shingles but likely genital herpes recurring on your buttocks. The next time you get those blisters, ask for a herpes simplex swab test, or you could ask for a herpes blood test now, if you prefer. I know this isn't good news, but at least it's factual news, and it may stimulate a discussion with your doctor that will help you get an effective treatment for this infection. By the way, the shingles vaccine doesn't treat shingles or herpes; its purpose is to prevent people from getting shingles. If you haven't had the vaccine already, I would advise that you get it. It is appropriate and advised for all adults age sixty and over.

About three weeks ago, I had sex several times over a weekend with someone new—no condoms. Yes, silly, I know. But I just had a herpes antibody test, and it's positive for HSV 2 at >5. Does this mean that my latest partner gave me herpes? This is my first herpes antibody test. I can't reach this person to get him tested to see if he has it. All you can determine from this antibody test is that you're infected. An antibody test can become positive as early as a week to ten days from infection, so you could've been infected by this person or by a partner from years ago. Now if you'd gotten a herpes antibody test three days after the sexual encounter and it was positive at >5, you'd know that you didn't just get infected but were infected at some earlier time. But in your situation, there's just no way to know how long you've had herpes.

Chapter 5

Special Concerns for Women: Protecting Yourself and Your Baby

Because women have unique internal genital parts that allow them to bear children and breastfeed, as well as subject them to the risk of developing cervical cancer, they get their own special chapter in this book. If you're a man, you should read it too, so you can appreciate what's up with your female partner.

HERPES INSIDE

So, what about those internal female parts—the cervix, vagina, uterus, and fallopian tubes—those parts you just can't see? How are they involved in herpes infection? We know that women can have outbreaks of herpes on the cervix and, sometimes though not often, inside the vagina. Remember that the cervix is that firm thing at the end of your vagina that feels like the tip of your nose. When outbreaks happen on the cervix, you obviously can't see them yourself, and quite honestly, if you have a speculum at home and are repeatedly examining your cervix to try to see lesions, you're way too caught up in your disease state.

It's quite common with first infection to have cervical involvement. As the cells of the cervix become infected, they break open and release their contents into the vagina, and you might notice a vaginal discharge that's typically clear to white and watery. I was involved in the case of a young woman whose first herpes outbreak was during late pregnancy.

She had enough discharge from the cervical involvement that she thought her bag of waters had sprung a significant leak!

Herpes lesions rarely occur on the vaginal walls beyond the opening to the vagina, and the disease doesn't move up inside the fallopian tubes or uterus and cause problems like scarring and infertility there, as gonorrhea and chlamydia can. So good—that's one less thing to worry about.

When the herpes virus reactivates, the cervix can become involved again, but there might not be any symptoms, even if you're shedding virus from that location. As we discussed earlier in the book, you can't know exactly when you're shedding virus, and that applies to both the inside and outside parts of your genitals, so you need to behave as though you could be shedding at any time from any of those places.

HERPES AND PREGNANCY

Pregnancy is a big concern for women who have herpes, and understandably so. Babies who get herpes at birth can be really sick and, in some cases, die. But if you recall reading earlier about how common genital herpes is and compare that to how uncommon neonatal herpes is, you should be greatly reassured. There's much that can be done to reduce the risk of neonatal herpes to levels that are very low indeed.

It's highly unusual for a baby to get infected while safely nestled in a closed sac during pregnancy. Most neonatal herpes happens during delivery, and that's where the focus of concern should be.

If you know you have genital herpes (whether type 1 or 2) and your provider knows it too, there's much less than a 1 percent chance that you'll infect your baby during pregnancy and delivery, and those are wonderful odds (Brown et al. 2003). It's essential, though, that your obstetric (OB) provider become aware of your herpes early in the pregnancy. A third to a fourth of all adult pregnant women have genital herpes (Xu et al. 2007), but almost 90 percent of them don't know they have it (Whitley, Davis, and Suppapanya 2007). A patient with genital herpes is not something new or shocking to your clinician, so don't be embarrassed to disclose your status. The fact that you and your clinician *do* know about it makes the situation much safer for your baby. I've known women who were so embarrassed about having herpes that they didn't tell their OB they were infected, and instead used hope and prayer as a method of reducing the risk of infecting their babies. That's not a wise decision, and I hope it's one you'll never make.

If you get pregnant while taking daily herpes medicine, it's not a problem at all. Most OB providers will ask you to stop daily therapy until close to the end of the pregnancy and just treat individual outbreaks if they come up. The outbreak treatment would last one to five days, depending on which medicine you take. If you have either type 1 or 2 genital infection, you'll probably be advised to begin taking daily antiviral therapy during the last weeks of your pregnancy. The purpose is twofold: it reduces the risk of having an outbreak at delivery that would necessitate a C-section, and it reduces viral shedding, which presents a risk to your baby during labor and delivery. Some OB providers start suppression at 32 weeks of gestation, others at 34 weeks, and most begin suppression at 36 weeks; all are reasonable choices. If you have or develop a condition that might require an early delivery—for example, if you're having twins or if you develop toxemia—suppression will likely be started earlier. The goal is to have had at least ten days of treatment in your system when the baby is delivered. The recommended dose is higher for pregnant women, because their immune systems are somewhat compromised by the pregnancy. The typical prescription is 500 milligrams of Valtrex (valacyclovir hydrochloride) twice daily or 400 milligrams of acyclovir three times daily late in pregnancy. Both are considered safe doses for the baby during pregnancy (Hollier and Wendel 2008; Sheffield et al. 2006).

Labor Precautions and Procedures

If you have the herpes virus and are pregnant, certain procedures will be avoided during labor. A fetal scalp electrode to monitor the baby's health probably won't be used, because it makes a small break in the baby's scalp skin that could allow entry of the herpes virus; rather, an external monitor will more likely be used to track the baby's status. Your membranes probably won't be intentionally ruptured early in the labor, because the bag of waters protects the baby from any herpes virus that might be in your genital area. The longer your membranes stay intact, the longer the baby benefits from this natural form of protection. If, during labor, your bag of waters has been broken for a long time, it's possible that your provider will become concerned about viral transmission to the baby and consider a C-section. Just be prepared to be flexible about that possibility. And be sure to continue your suppressive therapy throughout labor, right up until delivery.

If there's no herpes outbreak in your boxer-shorts area at delivery time, most OB providers will suggest that you have a vaginal delivery. But if there *is* an outbreak, it's wisest to have a C-section (ACOG 1999). Either way, the chances are excellent that you'll have a healthy baby.

Some HSV-positive readers will have pregnant female partners who are either currently uninfected or don't know their herpes status. Here's some guidance about HSV testing for women who are known to be uninfected or who are unsure about their herpes status.

Testing for Herpes in Pregnancy

Testing for herpes in pregnant women is controversial. However, there are two reasons why many experts now believe it's important to test all pregnant women for herpes infection. The first is to identify women who have herpes but don't know it so that the infection can be managed appropriately during pregnancy. The second is to identify uninfected women who could get genital herpes during the third trimester (Gardella and Brown 2007). Testing for other STIs in pregnancy is very common; most pregnant women are now routinely tested for gonorrhea, chlamydia, syphilis, and HIV. Oddly, HSV 2 infection is a more prevalent sexually transmitted infection than all the other STIs combined (CDC 2000), yet herpes testing of pregnant women is still uncommon and isn't yet recommended by the American College of Obstetricians and Gynecologists (1999).

If it's known that a pregnant woman has herpes, special care is taken during the pregnancy, and particularly during labor and delivery, to reduce the baby's risk of getting infected, but that special care can only be given when the woman is known to have herpes. That's why it's important to know which women are really infected, not just which women are aware of their infection.

If a woman gets either HSV 1 or 2 genital herpes for the first time during the third trimester of pregnancy, there's a 30 to 50 percent chance that she'll infect her baby (Kinghorn 2002; Gardella and Brown 2007). That's a high risk, isn't it? And here's why it's especially serious to get herpes during the third trimester of pregnancy and why it can happen more easily then as opposed to when a woman isn't pregnant:

- A pregnant woman is at a particularly higher risk of acquiring herpes, because her immune system is compromised by the pregnancy, which makes her more vulnerable to infection. For example, if a woman doesn't have either herpes type 1 or 2 and regularly has sex with an HSV 2 positive partner, there's a 19 percent chance she'll get HSV 2 from her partner during pregnancy (Brown et al. 1997).

- If she gets infected late in the pregnancy, her body has little time to make antibody and pass it to her baby prior to delivery, and it's important that the baby get antibody from the mom to help protect against possible infection.

- People with new genital herpes infection shed virus far more frequently than people with established infection (Wald et al. 2006b), and a pregnant woman is no exception; in fact, because her immune system is compromised, she may shed more virus with new infection than a woman who isn't pregnant.

The best way to diagnose herpes if you're pregnant is to get a type-specific blood antibody test eighteen to twenty-two weeks into the pregnancy or a little earlier in pregnancy, when blood is drawn. There are typically other blood tests drawn at eighteen to twenty-two weeks, so this is a convenient time to do the herpes testing. Doing the antibody test at this time in the pregnancy helps identify both those women who were infected before they got pregnant and those who became infected during the earlier weeks of pregnancy. It's critical to know before the beginning of the third trimester who's uninfected and, therefore, still vulnerable to infection, so couples can manage their sexual behavior to provide the greatest safety for their babies. Blood antibody testing begins with the mother. If her antibody test is positive for HSV 2, we already know what to do, and further testing is not required. Those protective measures for the baby are described earlier in this chapter. If the mother's blood antibody test is negative for both HSV 1 and 2, then she's vulnerable to acquiring HSV in the third trimester, which would not be good at all. There are two options available should she test negative for both HSV 1 and 2: her partner can be tested for antibody, or the couple can abstain from all sexual contact during the third trimester.

If the mother is found not to have herpes, and the couple wishes to continue sexual activity into the third trimester, antibody testing for the partner is the best approach and will give the couple the necessary information for how to proceed with their sex lives yet still protect their baby. If the mother has more than one partner, these principles apply to all of them.

Precautions Based on Each Partner's Herpes Status

The chart on the next page shows the best interventions for women and their partners based on the possible combination of antibody-test results. A plus sign (+) means a positive test result, and a minus sign (−) means a negative test result. "Doesn't matter" means that the test status doesn't make a difference to the baby's safety. Perhaps it goes without saying that if the mother or her partner has any other sexual partners during the pregnancy, the entire risk picture morphs into the unknown, which can be very risky for the baby.

Concerns About Herpes Testing in Pregnant Women

What are the concerns raised by testing for herpes in pregnancy? One is that finding out about a herpes infection during that delicate time of pregnancy is just too hard on couples and that relationships could suffer or be destroyed by the news. I agree that getting this news can be a challenge, but in a study of over seventy thousand women for whom herpes blood antibody testing was routinely done during pregnancy, Dr. Zane Brown and his colleagues (1991) found that the doomsday scenarios of couples getting divorced or violence happening within relationships simply didn't materialize. Couples should be informed that herpes infection can be present for many years before diagnosis occurs and that infidelity need not have happened for infection to be present. They also appreciate becoming aware of something that poses risks to the baby's health, even if the news means having to make adjustments in their sex lives.

Cost may be an obstacle to herpes testing for some women. Most private insurers cover herpes testing if the provider who orders the test

Pregnant Mother's Antibody Status	Partner's Antibody Status	Safety Precautions Necessary During Third Trimester
HSV 2 +; HSV 1 status doesn't matter.	No testing required for partner. Partner's status doesn't matter.	Standard precautions for a woman known to have recurrent genital herpes (discussed earlier).
HSV 1 and 2 -.	HSV 1 and 2 +.	Mother shouldn't receive oral sex from her partner, and they shouldn't have intercourse in the third trimester. This woman has the highest risk of getting infected from her partner.
HSV 1 and 2 -.	HSV 1 + with cold-sore history; HSV 2 -.	Mother shouldn't receive oral sex from her partner. Intercourse okay.
HSV 1 and 2 -.	HSV 1 + with no cold-sore history; HSV 2 -.	Mother shouldn't receive oral sex from or have intercourse with her partner.
HSV 1 + with history of cold sores; HSV 2 -.	HSV 1 +; HSV 2 -.	No precautions required for this couple.
HSV 1 + with no history of cold sores; HSV 2 -.	HSV 1 status doesn't matter; HSV 2 -.	No precautions for this couple, but the mother should be observed for any genital symptoms at delivery, in case her HSV 1 is genital.
HSV 1 + with or without cold-sore history; HSV 2 -.	HSV 1 status doesn't matter; HSV 2 +.	Best to avoid intercourse altogether during third trimester. If that's unacceptable, no unprotected intercourse in the third trimester. Partner should take suppression medication and use condoms if they do have intercourse. Receiving oral sex is okay for both partners.

feels it's necessary or desirable. For those patients who don't have insurance coverage for herpes testing, private payment for testing is an option. Several state programs provide pregnancy care, but most, unfortunately, don't pay for herpes testing. It's wise to consult the OB provider's office when issues of financial hardship are present.

Increased use of antiviral therapy in pregnant women is a concern that's been expressed by some clinicians. It's certain that if more women are diagnosed as having herpes when they're pregnant, more antiviral medication will be prescribed. But most OB providers believe that daily suppressive medication taken during the final few weeks of pregnancy is safe and effective for treating pregnant women infected with genital herpes. A similar concern is that if we start using antiviral therapy in larger populations of pregnant women, we might identify a side effect from the medication in newborns that we've not yet discovered. However, there's no data available that shows any increased risk of major birth defects in women treated with acyclovir during the first trimester of pregnancy, compared to the general population (Stone et al. 2004). This should reassure women who are worried about using antiviral therapy during pregnancy.

Another concern for health professionals is the time required for counseling pregnant women and their partners about newly diagnosed genital herpes infections. There's no doubt that those who test positive will require information and support, but much of that can be delivered through independent reading and video materials. Our goal should be to protect babies from possible infection, and all the obstacles to herpes testing during pregnancy are much easier to deal with than a case of neonatal herpes. Herpes testing in pregnancy will likely be an evolving issue in the coming years, so stay tuned.

Other Neonatal Transmission Risks

Genital herpes isn't the only risk for babies. After delivery, a few babies get infected with herpes from adults or older children who have cold sores and kiss them. Newborns simply lack an adequately developed immune system to deal with herpes viruses, so either HSV 1 or 2 can cause serious problems for a new arrival. It's the responsibility of parents and caregivers to be certain that no one with a cold sore ever kisses the baby while the baby's still small and vulnerable, specifically under six months of age. This is particularly true if the mother is HSV 1 negative and has never passed HSV 1 antibody to her baby during the pregnancy.

HERPES AND BREASTFEEDING

If you have genital herpes, you can definitely breastfeed, and breastfeeding provides your baby with a great head start to good health. There's only one thing about genital herpes that may restrict you. A few women do get herpes lesions on a breast, often contracted when someone with a cold sore put a mouth on a nipple, was a bit rough, and broke the skin, which allowed the virus in. If you've had outbreaks of herpes on a nipple, you should watch for outbreaks on the breast while nursing. If you experience an outbreak, pump and discard your milk, treat the outbreak, and resume nursing when the outbreak is over. Most OB providers and pediatricians don't restrict the use of antiviral therapy while nursing. Antiviral medicines do get into breast milk but only in insignificant amounts, and present no danger to the baby (Sheffield et al. 2002).

LIST OF QUESTIONS FOR PREGNANCY

If you have herpes and get pregnant, you'll certainly have lots of questions about how herpes impacts your pregnancy and what you should do about it during pregnancy and delivery. Below are some questions that might be useful to photocopy and take with you to your appointment. Providers tend to handle these issues in their own ways. What matters is that you feel confident and comfortable with the plan for your care.

If you have herpes, tell your OB provider about it and ask:

- How do you want me to handle any outbreaks that come up during my pregnancy?

- How will you manage my daily therapy at the end of pregnancy: when will I start treatment, what medicine will I take, and how much will I take per day?

- What special precautions will you take to protect my baby during labor and delivery?

- How do you feel about my taking herpes medication while breastfeeding?

- If I don't want to take any medication during pregnancy, what alternatives are available, if any?

- Under what circumstances would you recommend a C-section as it relates to my having herpes?

If you're reading this chapter because you're a woman whose partner has herpes but you don't, or if you don't know whether you have it and are planning to become pregnant or already are, ask your OB provider:

- Will I be tested for herpes, and if yes, when?

- If you don't do herpes testing, why not, and can I get tested some other way if I want to know if I'm infected?

- What precautions do you want me to take to avoid getting infected with herpes during my pregnancy?

- Should my infected partner be on daily therapy? Can you facilitate or prescribe that?

- What sexual behaviors should my partner and I avoid, if any?

HERPES AND CERVICAL CANCER

Some older studies suggested that herpes might be a cause of cervical cancer, but more-recent research has clearly identified human papillomavirus (HPV) as the culprit. HPV can be found in over 99 percent of cervical cancers (Wright et al. 2006), and evidence is growing that it's involved in rectal and oral cancers too (Hu and Goldie 2008). Certainly, if you're a woman with genital herpes, you should get regular Pap smears and evaluations for HPV. Be aware that the same behaviors that put you at risk for herpes type 2 also put you at risk for HPV infection, but you don't need to worry any more about your cervical-cancer risk increasing just because you have herpes. And when you're in for your Pap smear, talk with your clinician about the HPV vaccine that's available to reduce the risk of cervical cancer.

HERPES AND BIRTH CONTROL

Patients often ask if birth control pills have an impact on herpes recurrences. We've not seen any consistently documented connection between oral contraceptives and the frequency of herpes outbreaks or shedding. One study found somewhat increased shedding in women taking birth control pills (Cherpes et al. 2005), but another found no increase (Mohllajee et al. 2006), so the impact, if any, of oral contraceptives is somewhat unclear. Condoms obviously carry the dual benefit of birth control and some barrier protection against virus transmission. Female condoms may offer even more surface area coverage, but they haven't been studied as male condoms have.

QUESTIONS AND ANSWERS ABOUT WOMEN'S CONCERNS AND HERPES

I get a stringy discharge from my vagina about once a month around the middle of my menstrual cycle. Does that mean I'm having herpes outbreaks on my cervix? Research hasn't identified any particular time in the menstrual cycle when women have more herpes outbreaks or viral shedding. Though an individual woman might report herpes symptoms just before her period, just after, or midcycle, research hasn't found a particular time in the menstrual cycle when most women consistently have more herpes problems. Women ovulate in the middle of their menstrual cycles, and that can be accompanied by a stretchy, elastic discharge. A discharge caused by herpes on the cervix is quite watery, not stringy.

I'm thirty-seven weeks pregnant, taking 400 milligrams of acyclovir three times a day, and I'm not getting any outbreaks, but I still worry about asymptomatic viral shedding at the time of delivery. It seems as if this would still be an issue, or would it? It can be, but with daily suppressive medicine and careful observation for outbreaks, a vaginal delivery is still the preferred option for the best outcome. In studies where mothers were followed with daily genital swabbing close to delivery, even when shedding occurred and vaginal delivery happened, very few babies became infected (Sheffield et al. 2003). It appears that antibody transferred from mother to baby offers the greatest opportunity for protection. Expectant mothers and their medical providers must balance the risks of a C-section against the very low risk of infecting the baby.

I'm terrified that I'll infect my baby with herpes at delivery, so can I just get my doctor to do a C-section and not even attempt a vaginal delivery? You could ask. I'm sure your OB provider will take your fears into consideration along with the low medical risks of a C-section and the low likelihood that you would infect your baby. However, I encourage you to stay as flexible as possible, and continue to talk with your doctor about the options and take daily suppressive medicine at the end of your pregnancy. These medicines reduce the risk of herpes transmission from a mother to her baby to a negligible level. But do express your preferences; your feelings are an important part of the whole pregnancy process, and they matter very much.

After my annual exam last month, my nurse practitioner called and told me my Pap smear came back slightly abnormal—nothing major. I have herpes, and I think I was having an outbreak at the time of the exam. Could the herpes have caused the Pap to be abnormal, or is it for sure HPV? The HPV test that they did at the same time was negative. I'm not sure how to understand this, and neither was my nurse practitioner; she just said to come back in a year and we would do it again. It's possible that having a herpes outbreak on the cervix at the time of your Pap could cause your Pap to look abnormal, especially since the HPV part of the lab work was negative. Sometimes a Pap smear will pick up herpes-infected cells, and that will appear on the report, but I think, this time, it didn't show that specifically. I would follow your nurse practitioner's advice and get the testing redone in a year to see what comes up. It's good that the HPV test was negative at this time.

I have frequently recurring cold sores but not genital herpes. Do I need to take daily therapy at the end of my pregnancy too? No, you don't, but if you get a cold sore when your baby is small, be sure not to kiss the baby until the cold sore is healed. And don't let grandparents or anyone else with a cold sore kiss your baby either. If a newborn baby gets the cold-sore virus from an adult, it can be life threatening.

Chapter 6

Treatment and Vaccines: The Really Good News

So you've confirmed your herpes diagnosis with the appropriate lab tests, you're working on accepting "the news," and now you're wondering about treatment options. A little background information will help.

THE HERPES MEDICINES

Did you know that as recently as 1981, there was no treatment for herpes? You may not have even been born yet, or you may have been diagnosed before that year. Back then, a genital herpes diagnosis came with instructions to just wait out every outbreak, along with the bad news that there was nothing to help reduce the frequency of recurrences. You were told that only using condoms and avoiding sex during outbreaks could reduce the risk of transmission to others. What frustration and feelings of hopelessness often followed! Thankfully, we're in a new era, and we now have three drugs that are effective in treating genital and oral herpes, as well as some very promising ones that are now in clinical development.

Antivirals vs. Antibiotics

Since herpes is a virus, the medications used to treat it are antivirals. Antivirals aren't the same as antibiotics. Antibiotics are used to treat bacterial infections, and antivirals, like the ones we've been discussing, are used to treat viral infections. The following chart compares their differences.

	ANTIBIOTICS	ANTIVIRALS
Treats	Bacterial infections	Viral infections
Purpose	Cures the infection	Only treats infection rather than curing disease
The body develops resistance to the medicine over time	Quite common	Very uncommon (except with some HIV medicines)
Importance of finishing all the pills	Very important	Not important
Use continuing over several years on a daily basis	Uncommon	Common

In 1982, acyclovir, the first of the oral antiviral medications, became available by prescription. (A little history: Acyclovir was developed by Gertrude Elion, the daughter of immigrant Jewish parents living in New York City. Trudy, as she was affectionately known, graduated from high school at age fifteen and from Hunter College at nineteen. She then met and became engaged to Leonard Canter. They were both scientists with amazing futures ahead, but Leonard developed endocarditis, an infection of the heart, in the days before penicillin was discovered. He died within six months, and no one ever recaptured Trudy's heart. Instead, she pursued her Ph.D. at night while working during the day for Burroughs Wellcome and Company, collaborating with George Hutchings, Ph.D. Trudy had a master's degree, but in her field, a Ph.D. was really the minimum standard to become a noted academic scientist. The dean of her Ph.D. program told her to make a choice: either pursue the degree full-time during the day and quit her job, or discontinue her Ph.D. program. Her decision to stay in pharmaceutical research with just her master's degree in hand led to the development of several groundbreaking drugs and, eventually, the 1988 Nobel Prize in Medicine for her work.)

There are now three antivirals available in the United States:

- **acyclovir** (also known by the brand name Zovirax)

- **valacyclovir** (also known by the brand name Valtrex)

- **famciclovir** (also known by the brand name Famvir)

All fall into a category called *nucleoside analogs*, and function in pretty much the same way. Because viruses require certain nutrients in order to live and reproduce, these medicines present themselves to the virus as one of the nutrients it needs, but they're really just pretenders. When the virus takes up the pretender medicine to make more DNA to reproduce, it can't do it, because the look-alike nutrient isn't the real thing. The virus doesn't die off completely, but its replication is temporarily and greatly slowed down so that outbreaks resolve and shedding is reduced.

Though acyclovir was a huge step from no treatment at all, it turned out that only about 15 percent of the medicine inside each pill was available for the body to use. In medical lingo, that's called *poor bioavailability*, and means that the medicine needs to be taken quite often to work well.

Then came valacyclovir, which is a better-absorbed and utilized version of acyclovir. Because of its chemical structure, the body can use a whole lot more of the medicine in valacyclovir, so it can be taken a lot less often than acyclovir. When it passes through the liver, it's changed into acyclovir. This is good, because we know a lot about acyclovir; it's been around for quite a while, it's safe, and it works well.

Around the same time, famciclovir was developed. It has a slightly different structure but works in a similar way, and also has high bioavailability, requiring less frequent dosing. Acyclovir and famciclovir are both available in generic form; valacyclovir will be available as a generic in December 2009.

First-Outbreak Treatment

It's wise to treat the first outbreak, when symptoms are usually more difficult, because treatment really helps the outbreak resolve more quickly and reduces the amount of time spent shedding or giving off virus (Fife et al. 1997). Sometimes people with first infections initially have mild symptoms but, after five days or so, get a whole new batch of sores. Taking medicine can often keep that second round from happening. You might also have difficulty urinating and sometimes experience a splitting headache or sensitivity to light, and taking medicine can help keep these first-outbreak symptoms under control. In the table below, I've listed the CDC's recommended doses for the first outbreak for all three drugs (2006). You'll notice that these doses are considerably higher than those to treat subsequent outbreaks or to be taken daily.

Recommended Doses For First Outbreak

acyclovir (Zovirax)	400 mg three times a day for 7 to 10 days *or* 200 mg five times a day for 7 to 10 days
valacyclovir (Valtrex)	1,000 mg (1 gram) twice a day for 7 to 10 days
famciclovir (Famvir)	250 mg three times per day for 7 to 10 days

When writing prescriptions to treat a suspected first outbreak, many clinicians make a refill available, because patients often don't feel that they're quite over their symptoms within ten days. If you're having a first outbreak right now and need more days of medicine, don't hesitate to ask your clinician for a refill. You'll notice that with acyclovir, there are two different dose schedules listed. Some people might want to take fewer doses during the day, because they aren't good at remembering to take pills. The second option calls for more-frequent dosing with smaller amounts of medicine. Clinicians might assume that everyone wants to take less-frequent doses, but I've worked with many patients who *want* to take doses more frequently, because it feels as if they're actively doing something about their outbreaks throughout the day. You should base how you take the medicine on your personal lifestyle and your clinician's recommendations. The two schedules are equally effective.

Deciding What to Do Next

Let's say that your first outbreak is over and you've got some decisions to make. Will you now take medicine every day, will you treat outbreaks as they come up, or will you forgo treatment altogether and wait to see how you do? The following flow chart shows your choices.

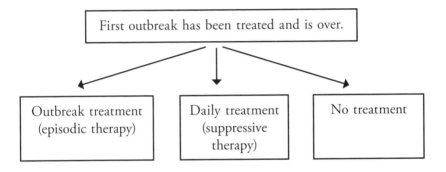

Here are some things we know about what happens after that first outbreak:

- People diagnosed with untreated genital HSV 2 have an average of four to six recurrences in the first year, and 20 percent have ten or more recurrences per year (Benedetti, Corey, and Ashley 1994). Genital HSV 1 recurs much less often than HSV 2.

- People who have a new infection (which a positive swab test and a negative antibody test for the same type of virus will reveal) shed virus on about 41 percent of days of the first few months of infection (Gupta et al. 2004). Some of that shedding will happen during symptoms, and some will happen without symptoms. That means that newly infected people are considerably more infectious to others than those who've been infected longer.

- Newly infected people often experience psychological upset regarding the diagnosis, but almost all bounce back to baseline psychological functioning within four to six months (Rosenthal et al. 2006; Miyai et al. 2004). However, those who start taking medication daily right away have better psychological adjustment than those who don't (Handsfield et al. 2007).

Suppressive Therapy

Suppressive therapy means that you take herpes medicine every day. All three medicines have been shown to reduce the frequency of outbreaks and extend the amount of time between them (CDC 2006). The following table shows the doses that are effective for daily therapy for the three medicines.

EFFECTIVE DOSES FOR DAILY THERAPY

acyclovir (Zovirax)	400 mg twice a day
valacyclovir (Valtrex)	500 mg once a day if you have nine or fewer outbreaks per year *or* 1,000 mg (1 gram) once a day if you have ten or more outbreaks a year
famciclovir (Famvir)	250 mg twice a day

These are the recommended doses, but they aren't written in stone. You may need a little more medicine to keep your herpes quiet, or you might get by on even less medicine than the recommended dose. You may benefit from breaking up the doses more frequently over the course of the day. The doses listed on the chart are your starting place, and there's room here to be flexible enough to meet your individual needs. Work with your clinician to figure out what dose and frequency works best for you.

Benefits of Suppressive Therapy: Taking antiviral medicine on a daily basis reduces the frequency of herpes outbreaks, reduces viral shedding, and reduces the risk of infecting a sex partner (Reitano et al. 1998; Corey et al. 2004). When taken as directed, all three medicines work equally well. The differences between them are frequency of dosing, cost, and insurance coverage. Both acyclovir and famciclovir are taken twice daily, while valacyclovir is taken only once a day. Taking any of the three antiviral medicines daily (compared to a placebo, such as a sugar pill or another inactive substance) reduces the frequency of recurrences by about 70 to 80 percent and reduces viral shedding by 80 to 94 percent, and valacyclovir reduces the chance of infecting a sexual partner by 48 percent.

Candidates for Suppressive Therapy: Is suppressive therapy right for you? Go through this list to see if any of these situations fits yours. If suppressive therapy doesn't seem right for you, then maybe outbreak therapy would be better; that list comes a little later in the chapter.

You have an uninfected partner. A study following almost fifteen hundred discordant couples (one partner is infected, and the other is not) found a 48 percent reduction in transmission when the infected partners took 500 milligrams of valacyclovir (Valtrex) daily (Corey et al. 2004). Cutting transmission in half clearly isn't perfection, but think of it as one tool in the toolbox; it's one strategy that, when combined with others (like condom use and symptom awareness), provides a very good reduction in risk. If you're infected and your partner isn't, and you both agree that transmission reduction is something you want to shoot for, then daily therapy can be a big part of the solution.

You have more than one partner, not all of whom have been tested to determine if they're infected. However, you'd like to do what you can to reduce the risk of giving people herpes, if they happen to be uninfected.

You're bothered by herpes outbreaks. You don't have to have lots of outbreaks for them to be bothersome, but it's a very individual matter. More than ten outbreaks a year might be the intolerable point for one person, and for another, it might be two. There's no magic number of outbreaks that indicates the need for suppression. It's up to you to decide how important this issue is, but daily therapy will reduce the frequency of recurrences for almost everyone who takes antiviral medicine. But remember, herpes isn't just about outbreaks; it's also about viral shedding and the risk it poses to uninfected partners.

You're newly infected with genital herpes. Suppression provides clear benefits for the person who's had a genital herpes outbreak for the first time. You'll see more about this a little farther along in this chapter.

You're late in a late stage of pregnancy. As we discussed in detail in chapter 5, most pregnant women who have herpes benefit from daily therapy starting at thirty-two to thirty-six weeks and continuing through delivery. Treatment reduces the risk of having an outbreak at the time of delivery, which would otherwise necessitate having a C-section. Treatment also reduces viral shedding at delivery time for greater safety of the baby (Sheffield et al. 2006; Hollier and Wendel 2008).

Suppressive Therapy Early in Infection: We know that in the early months of infection, people experience the most outbreaks, the most viral shedding, and the most emotional upset. In the past, however, prescribing daily therapy was postponed until some arbitrary benchmark was met, usually when some specific number of outbreaks had occurred. But looking back, waiting didn't make much sense.

Two research studies evaluated starting people who have new genital HSV 2 on daily suppressive therapy immediately after diagnosis and after the first-episode treatment was finished. I'm fortunate to have been an author on both of those papers, and what we found was that people on antiviral therapy (in this case, valacyclovir) had significantly fewer outbreaks than those on a placebo (Fife et al. 2008) and that their psychological adjustment was also better on medicine than a placebo (Handsfield et al. 2007). If you're newly diagnosed with HSV 2, you may wish to consider daily therapy for six to twelve months, as you get used to having herpes. If you want to just wait to see how things go without further treatment, that's okay too. If you decide not to take daily treatment now, you can always change your mind and ask later for the prescription for daily therapy.

Outbreak (Episodic) Therapy

Outbreak therapy, also known as *episodic therapy*, is taking medicine only when you have an outbreak. If you take medicine at the start of an outbreak, you decrease viral shedding, reduce pain, and speed healing of the outbreak by about one to two days (Bodsworth et al. 1997). If your outbreaks last five days (which is usual), then that's a 20 percent improvement. But if your outbreaks last two weeks, a one-day to two-day reduction isn't that great. Dosing for outbreak therapy has changed a lot since we started using these medicines. Early on, the recommended dosing schedules required several days of treatment, but more recently, studies have found that only a day or two of treatment is just as effective (Aoki et al. 2006; Bavaro et al. 2008, Wald et al. 2002). Following are suggested doses for episodic therapy for genital herpes.

SUGGESTED DOSES OF ORAL ANTIVIRALS FOR EPISODIC THERAPY

Acyclovir	Valacyclovir	Famciclovir
400 mg three times a day for five days *or* 800 mg twice a day for five days *or* 800 mg three times a day for two days	500 mg twice a day for three days *or* 1,000 mg (1 gram) once a day for five days *or* 2,000 mg (2 grams) twice a day for one day	1,000 mg twice a day for one day *or* 125 mg twice daily for five days

Candidates for Outbreak Therapy: Is episodic therapy right for you? See how this list of situations fits you.

> **You have infrequent outbreaks that don't last very long and don't bother you much when they happen.** This might be because you have HSV 1 genital infection; remember that it recurs genitally less often than HSV 2.

You're not very good at taking pills every day. This may be either because you have trouble remembering or you don't like taking medicines that often, especially when there are no symptoms.

Your partner is infected with the same type of herpes simplex virus that you are, and you aren't bothered enough by your outbreaks to take medicine every day. If you're both infected with HSV 1 or you're both infected with HSV 2, then there's little need to worry anymore about genital herpes transmission in your sexual relationship. You can have sex when it's comfortable for both of you. There's no concern about triggering more outbreaks or passing the virus back and forth between you and your partner.

You're not sexually active right now. In this case, there's no risk of infecting someone else, and you aren't bothered by your outbreaks enough to take medicine every day.

Episodic Therapy for Oral Herpes: The episodic therapy doses for oral herpes are a bit different. Oral herpes outbreaks progress from prodromal symptoms to a full-blown outbreak very quickly, so a higher dose of medicine over a shorter period of time is required to treat the outbreak (Gilbert 2007). Effective doses for treating cold-sore outbreaks are 1,500 milligrams of famciclovir in a single dose on one day only, or 2,000 milligrams of valacyclovir twice on one day only.

Episodic Suppression

There's a gray area between taking medication daily and treating outbreaks as they come up. Episodic suppression means taking daily medicine for some extended period of time for a specific reason. You might want to use this treatment method for the following reasons (and maybe others that you can think of):

- You're getting married, and you don't want a cold sore on your lip for the wedding pictures (if you have oral outbreaks) or a genital herpes outbreak during the honeymoon trip.

- You're having a cosmetic surgery procedure done on your face, and you don't want a cold sore complicating the healing process, since the procedure could trigger an outbreak. Trauma to the facial or genital nerve group is enough to trigger an outbreak in some people. The same could apply to back surgery, which could trigger a genital herpes outbreak.

- Treatment at the end of pregnancy is a form of episodic suppression; you're trying to reduce viral shedding and reduce the risk of getting an outbreak, which would require a C-section.

- You're cramming for an important exam, staying up late at night, and feeling very stressed. The last thing you need is to have to deal with a herpes outbreak.

You get the picture. However, a little planning is helpful. Whether you want to take suppression either episodically or all the time, about five days are needed for the medicine to become fully effective. In other words, if you've got a special liaison planned for Friday night, and want the best odds to prevent an outbreak and reduce viral shedding, start taking your medication on Sunday, not Thursday night.

Side Effects of Oral Medicines

The uncommon side effects with this group of three antiviral medicines are headache and nausea. In those taking the medicine suppressively, these side effects happened only slightly more often to study participants who took the active drug than to those who took a placebo (Tyring, Baker, and Snowden 2002). If you experience either of these problems, you could cut down the dose and take smaller amounts at first. Then, if you tolerate that, gradually increase the dose to the optimally effective level. Most people who initially experience these side effects get over them after taking the drug for a short time. Allergies to this class of drug are also very rare, but if you have any unusual symptoms after beginning to take any of the three antiviral medicines, notify your clinician.

Safety and Long-Term Use

Acyclovir has been in use since 1982 and, since that time, has been shown to be very safe. There's no evidence of kidney or liver problems associated with this class of drug, and studies haven't found any danger in continuing to take it over a long period of time (Tyring, Baker, and Snowden 2002).

Resistance

With antibiotic therapy, clinicians are concerned about resistance. That's when bacteria mutate and become unresponsive to the effects of the medication. There's a genuine concern about the so-called "super-bugs" that have become unresponsive to most or all antibiotics. But remember, herpes is a virus, not a bacterium, and so far, we've seen very little of this problem with the herpes medicines. Resistance is rarely seen, and only about 0.3 percent, or about one in a thousand, of all herpes virus strains in healthy people are resistant to the medicines available (Danve-Szatanek et al. 2004). Some of these strains are seen in people who've taken medicine, and some aren't. And sometimes during an outbreak, a person will give off a strain of virus that's resistant and then, with the very next outbreak, give off a strain of virus that's completely susceptible to herpes medicines.

Some strains of herpes virus lack a chemical necessary to allow the antiviral medicines to work. People who have compromised immune systems, such as those who are HIV positive or have AIDS, do have higher rates of resistance, because the virus can mutate more easily in people whose immune systems are already compromised.

Treating the Uninfected Partner

I'm often asked if there's a benefit to treating the uninfected partner in a discordant couple. The answer is, not usually. There are a few circumstances, however, when this might be helpful. Let's say that a known discordant couple is having intercourse and the infected partner is using a condom that breaks. The couple notices the start of an outbreak beneath the condom they hadn't noticed before. It might be beneficial for the uninfected partner to take relatively high doses of antiviral medicine— for example, 1 gram of Valtrex three or four times a day for three or four days—to try to prevent the virus from establishing itself in the boxer-shorts nerve group. Another time when it might be helpful to treat the uninfected partner is after a sexual assault. To be useful—and we really don't know if it would be—it must be done right away, within a couple of hours of the unexpected herpes virus exposure. After that amount of time, the virus would've had a good chance to find a home in the nerve group of the uninfected person. So there's little downside of experimentally treating the uninfected partner, except perhaps the cost. This treatment option is even discussed in the bulletin of the rather conservative American College of Obstetricians and Gynecologists (1999), so it isn't that wild of an idea.

Topical Antiviral Medicines

There are three topical antiviral medicines approved to treat herpes simplex infections. Acyclovir cream has been around for many years, and you might think that it would be a good supplement or even a replacement for oral medicine. It turns out, however, that treating genital herpes with topical medicine offers little, if any, benefit, and the CDC no longer recommends it. Denavir is a prescription topical form of famciclovir that's FDA approved for the treatment of cold sores. It shortens the duration of a fever blister by about a day. Abreva is an over-the-counter topical treatment for cold sores that offers a slight reduction in the duration of an outbreak.

There are some topical medicines you definitely should avoid. While steroid creams are useful for treating certain skin rashes, they're bad for treating genital herpes. They take away the skin's immune response that's necessary to resolve an outbreak, and patients who've mistakenly used steroid creams to treat their herpes have inadvertently kept their outbreaks going for weeks!

In general, when thinking about topical treatment, remember that the herpes virus likes to replicate where it's warm and wet, so your goal should be to keep the outbreak area cool and dry. Any topical medicine that keeps the area moist, such as creams and ointments, can work against you.

Treatments That Need Further Study

Resiquimod, a topical medicine, is an *immune-modulator drug*, meaning that the medicine encourages the immune system to respond more effectively to a problem. Its sister drug, imiquimod (also known by the brand name Aldara), has shown good success in treating genital warts and several other skin conditions. One study showed some limited benefit for treating genital herpes while using resiquimod, but more research will help clarify its degree of usefulness (Mark et al. 2007).

There's also a class of drugs called *helicase-primase inhibitors* that's currently being studied, but at this writing there's no data on the success of these medicines.

Other Treatments

There are things you can do to cope with genital herpes that don't involve prescription medicines. These might include comfort measures for your genitals during outbreaks, or activities that can help with your emotions, such as taking stress-reduction technique classes, exercising to get the endorphins going, getting relaxation or meditation training, receiving a massage, or undergoing counseling to start feeling more comfortable in your own skin. Your clinician may be able to recommend someone in your community for you to talk to, or give you the number of a local support group. We'll talk more about psychological interventions in chapter 8. The basics are to eat well, exercise often, get plenty of sleep, make friends, stay close to your family, and learn to be as happy as you can be. These life choices can't help but give your immune system a boost.

Ineffective Treatments

Although the following treatments have been discussed over the years as possible interventions for genital herpes, research hasn't shown them to have any positive effect in preventing or treating herpes outbreaks.

- Bacillus Calmette-Guérin (BCG) vaccine
- BHT
- Chloroform
- Ether
- Glossypol
- Influenza vaccine
- Lithium succinate cream
- Lysine

- Neutral red dye with light activation

- Proflavine

- Polio vaccine

- Smallpox vaccine (may even be harmful)

Lysine: Let's talk a little more about lysine, because it's a common amino acid that many people use to treat herpes. About forty years ago, some preliminary research indicated that this amino acid helped to slow the growth of herpes virus in the lab. The problem is that well-controlled studies on humans don't show a benefit from taking lysine. However, if you take lysine and see a benefit, then there's probably no downside to taking it except the expense. A "competing" amino acid is arginine, and the old thinking was that if lysine helped slow herpes growth, then arginine made herpes grow more. So for a long time, people avoided foods high in arginine, like chocolate and nuts, believing that they'd make their herpes worse, but that has never been proven either. So people have been unnecessarily avoiding chocolate for years, and that's a real shame!

Internet Products: There are other products, promoted primarily on the Internet, that aren't listed here. They're too numerous to count, and most will likely be gone as quickly as they appeared. You've heard the saying, "If it seems too good to be true, it probably is." Well, that definitely applies to the vast majority of products listed on the Internet as treatments and cures for genital herpes. Everyone who has herpes would love a cure, right? So there's always a disreputable person just a click away, ready to prey on that desire. But when there actually *is* a cure for herpes, it won't be found for $69.99 on the Internet; it will be featured in the lead article in the *New England Journal of Medicine*.

Symptom Relief

There's a wide range of symptoms that people can have with their genital herpes. Your outbreaks may cause you significant pain, or you may only notice some mild itching or irritation. The person who has very painful outbreaks may have trouble imagining that someone else might have little recognition that an outbreak is even present, but the truth is that the severity of symptoms varies widely among individuals. If you feel the need for symptom relief, I've listed some suggestions below. They certainly aren't cures, and they haven't been researched in clinical trials, but patients tell me that these measures help them feel more comfortable when they get outbreaks.

Spray Anesthetic Pain Relievers: Pain-relieving topical sprays are probably the most widely used treatment for herpes (other than antiviral therapy). Sprays are quite nice, because they can be applied without touching the skin, which could cause more pain. Using a spray also reduces the fear that touching the lesion could somehow move the virus around to another part of the body (usually an unfounded fear as long as hands have been washed). The spray is applied to the skin, and the nerve endings it touches are temporarily numbed, resulting in temporary pain relief. These products are typically sold to people to relieve sunburn pain, hemorrhoids, and other skin problems, and herpes pain usually isn't listed on the label. When trying to locate these products, look for something ending in "-caine" on the ingredient label, such as "lidocaine" or "xylocaine." A small number of people who use these sprays experience skin irritation, but that's unusual. You can find these products over the counter in any pharmacy, and when you buy one, no one will have a clue what you're buying it for. They're inexpensive and simple to use.

You might want a quick spray just before urinating, if your lesions are in a place that urine touches as it passes over the area, which can sting. If you don't get adequate pain relief from over-the-counter products, you can ask your clinician for a stronger version in prescription form.

Urinating Into Water: For women in particular, urination can be a real problem. When lesions are present, the nerves are raw and exposed, and urine is acidic, so the combination can be painful. There are a few ways to help this situation. One is to get a sitz-bath tub that accommodates your bottom, and you can find one at most pharmacies. Fill the tub with water, and right before you have to pee, immerse your entire genital area in the water. When urine hits the water, it's immediately diluted, greatly decreasing the burning sensation. Another strategy is to get a squirt bottle, and squirt the water over your genitals as you urinate into the toilet. The principle is the same: dilute the urine immediately to reduce the burning.

Loose Clothing: Long, flowing skirts (without underwear) and loose boxer shorts are "high fashion" for outbreak times. These items of clothing allow air to circulate freely around the genitals and help keep the cloth from touching tender, open lesions. If underwear is necessary, try to use those made from cotton, rather than synthetic, fibers so the fabric can "breathe."

Drying Agents: Drying agents include such products as Burrows Solution, which speeds the drying of lesions by absorbing excess moisture from the skin. Remember that the herpes virus likes to be wet and warm to replicate, so keeping the area cool and dry can speed healing. These agents come in a package with instructions for preparation. Usually, they're dissolved in a specific quantity of water in a sitz bath, described earlier. People with hemorrhoids or recent stitches from childbirth also use these sitz-bath tubs, so you don't even need to worry about pharmacy personnel associating them with genital herpes. Since soaking can be overdone, you'll want to limit the amount of time that you sit in the water to about fifteen minutes, twice a day.

Tannic Acid: Tannic acid, found in black tea, helps some people to reduce the itching and pain associated with an outbreak. A moistened, cool tea bag can be placed directly against the lesion for a pleasant cooling effect.

Ice: Remember how the herpes virus likes to be warm? When applied directly to the area of the outbreak and used during prodrome, ice may abort or slow down an outbreak for some people. You can put cracked ice in a small plastic bag, tie off the end securely, and wrap the bag in a thin towel. Put it inside your underwear to hold it in place. You can also try putting ice packs on your lip if you feel a cold sore coming on.

Vaccines

There are two kinds of vaccines: one is *prophylactic* (designed to protect people from getting herpes), while the other is *therapeutic* (designed to help people who already have herpes). When you normally think of vaccines, you only think about the prophylactic kind. You get a tetanus vaccination to keep from getting tetanus, right? But now, studies are under way to see if a vaccine can help you more effectively fight an infection; that's called a *therapeutic vaccine*.

A *prophylactic vaccine* to protect against getting HSV 2 is currently being tested in the United States (Stanberry et al. 2002). It's a *subunit recombinant vaccine*, which means that it contains only a small portion of the virus's genetic material. The vaccine has been effective only for women, not men, and it's only effective (if, in fact, the studies confirm it to be effective) for women who are antibody negative for both HSV 1 and 2. A very large-scale trial involving this vaccine started in 2003 (Stanberry et al. 2002). It won't help the person who already has herpes but, if proven effective, will be useful for those who want to lessen their chances of contracting herpes.

There are also early therapeutic vaccine trials ongoing for those already infected with HSV 2. The goal of a therapeutic vaccine is to enhance the body's immune response to herpes to decrease the frequency of shedding and outbreaks.

We anxiously await the progress of these vaccine trials. Three prophylactic vaccine trials have already been conducted that failed, but we hope that in the future, medical technology will offer something much better. Stay tuned.

QUESTIONS AND ANSWERS ABOUT HERPES TREATMENT

I've had genital herpes for a long time, and I used to have a great job with health insurance, so I took Valtrex once daily for suppression because that was covered under my plan. Now I've lost that job and honestly can't afford to pay out of pocket for Valtrex anymore. What can I do? There are a couple of options: You could switch to generic acyclovir, but you'll need to remember to take it twice a day rather than once. With a little discipline, you can make that change. Many pharmacy chains now offer four-dollar prescriptions for certain medications, and acyclovir is on that list at certain doses. You can probably get a month of suppression for around twelve dollars with acyclovir, and 400 milligrams twice a day should work about the same as Valtrex if you take it regularly, which is the key. If your income is low enough, you may qualify for some of the prescription-drug patient-assistance plans offered through GlaxoSmithKline's website (www.valtrex.com) or your clinician. (More Web addresses are provided in chapter 11).

I take Valtrex every day, and I don't have outbreaks anymore. I've never told my current partner that I have herpes, because my medicine works so well. It's difficult to say anything about it now, and frankly I don't see any reason to because of the success of my treatment. Is this okay? No, I don't think it is okay. Partners need to know that you have herpes so that they can make choices about risking infection and get tested to see if they're infected already. Though your medicine is working to keep outbreaks away, it's not perfect at reducing shedding. You can still infect others, even though you're not having symptoms. I know it's difficult to talk about herpes, but the trust between the two of you is dependent upon sharing important information, and this is certainly important. At this point, I think you could explain that you were confused about the need to tell partners about your herpes because your medicine was keeping outbreaks away, but you've recently learned that having no outbreaks doesn't mean that there's no possibility of transmission. It may also help to read chapter 8 to learn how to tell your partner that you have herpes. If your relationship is strong, I bet mutual understanding will prevail in the long run, even if there may be some hurt feelings in the short run.

I was diagnosed with HSV 2 genital infection about five years ago and had been having about four outbreaks a year. I was just treating them as they came up, because they only lasted a few days and my husband also has HSV 2. I didn't see any point in taking daily medicine, but about six months ago I started getting outbreaks every month that last almost two weeks each time. I told my ob-gyn about it, so she tested me for HIV infection and did some other blood tests to see if my immune system was functioning okay. That was scary, but everything was negative. Then she put me on daily suppressive therapy with 250 milligrams of famciclovir twice a day. I took it religiously for three months, but it's made no difference in the frequency of my outbreaks. If anything, they're lasting longer. I'm getting desperate! What can I do? I recommend that you go back to square one. You had herpes for several years with a completely normal recurrence pattern, but now you're in a very different place, symptomwise. One of the mistakes clinicians make with herpes is deciding that if someone tests positive for HSV 2, then everything happening in the genital area of that person *is* herpes. It's important to remember, however, that people with genital herpes can have other kinds of genital issues going on, and my suspicion is that you fall into that group. Your immune system was fine, but all of a sudden your recurrence pattern changed and suppression made no impact on your outbreaks. Those two things together suggest that your symptoms are caused by something else. Please return to your ob-gyn and ask him or her to consider other causes for your symptoms.

I was diagnosed with genital HSV 1 by a swab test from a group of sores about six months ago. I was put on 400 milligrams of acyclovir, twice a day, right away. I've been taking it ever since, but I still have daily symptoms of herpes in my genital area. I'm wondering if I should switch to a different medicine. Your case is a bit similar to the previous one. Just because a person is diagnosed with herpes doesn't mean that herpes causes all symptoms in the genital area. In your case, that's especially true since you have HSV 1 genital infection. HSV 1 recurs infrequently in the genital area, so symptoms that occur there every day and aren't impacted by medication probably aren't caused by the HSV 1 infection. Make another appointment to see what's really going on down there, so you can start getting treated with something appropriate to your condition.

I'm not a prescription-medicine kind of guy. Generally, I prefer naturopathic or homeopathic kinds of treatment. If I don't take one of the prescription antivirals, will my herpes get worse? And do you know of a proven natural treatment for herpes? I'm not sexually active right now, but I'm having outbreaks about every other month and would like to try something. The first answer is no; your herpes will take its normal course, whether or not you treat it, and won't get worse. However, I'm not aware of any nonprescription treatment that's been shown in recognized, controlled studies to be effective in treating herpes. I'm a "science-y" kind of clinician who doesn't really recommend unproven treatments to patients. But I'm guessing that you have a naturopathic or homeopathic provider who may have seen you for other things. Why not ask that person for some ideas? You've really got nothing to lose if what your alternative provider recommends is reputable and safe. The problem with alternative treatments is that large studies haven't been done to prove whether or not they really work. If John, from down the street, says a homegrown cream of garlic and goldenseal applied to his lesions resolves them within two days, we have no idea if that would work for other people unless a study is done on hundreds of people that compares it to a placebo cream. But who would fund that study? You can see the problem, I'm sure.

I take 200 milligrams of acyclovir once a day, which keeps me from getting outbreaks, so why would I want to take 400 milligrams twice a day? There are two basic reasons why people take daily herpes medicine: one is to reduce the frequency of outbreaks, and the other is to reduce the risk of infecting a partner. While 200 milligrams of acyclovir may prevent you from getting outbreaks, if you have a sexual partner or may have one in the future who's at risk of getting herpes, the dose of medicine you're on isn't enough, or taken often enough, to adequately impact viral shedding. Maybe you can take the 200 milligrams once a day while you don't have an at-risk partner, but go up to the 400 milligrams twice a day when you do. As mentioned before, viral shedding and outbreaks aren't the same thing, and shedding can happen between outbreaks.

There are so many suspicious offerings on the Internet to treat and cure herpes. Doesn't the FDA or some other governmental agency regulate these claims? "Natural products," such as food supplements and other items of this kind, aren't regulated in the same way that prescription medicines are. However, recently the FDA has cracked down on several sites offering herpes cures and made them pull some of their claims about the ability to cure herpes. Unfortunately, more may pop up tomorrow, but at least there's some action being taken.

I've been on suppressive therapy for one year, and now my doctor says I have to come off of therapy. Before the daily pills, I had outbreaks every single month, and now I have about one per year. The idea of going back to that old pattern stresses me out. What's the prevailing opinion about long-term therapy? Most clinicians would agree to keep patients on daily therapy for years. No side effects have been noted in patients who've taken these medicines for extended periods of time (Tyring, Baker, and Snowden 2002). We see no lab abnormalities associated with this drug and very little resistance (discussed earlier in this chapter).

I'm on suppressive therapy, but I'm unclear about how long I should be taking it: for a year, ten years, the rest of my life? Studies have shown that long-term therapy with acyclovir is safe and remains effective over time (Tyring, Baker, and Snowden 2002); the two other drugs haven't been around as long, but there's no reason to believe they're any different. Whether or not you want to continue the medicine depends on your situation; for example, if you have an uninfected partner, you'll want to avoid outbreaks, reduce shedding, and so on. I've had patients on daily therapy for twenty years, and they simply don't want to come off. The decision about long-term therapy should be based on your personal situation and preferences.

I didn't treat my first outbreak of herpes. At first, I didn't know what was going on, and by the time I figured it out a week later, it was starting to heal. I didn't have the money to buy the prescription that I was given, so the outbreak just healed on its own. Am I going to have more outbreaks in the future because I didn't treat the first one? No studies have been done to determine whether failure to treat a first outbreak has any impact on future outbreaks. Treating a first outbreak just makes you more comfortable faster.

I don't have genital herpes, but I have frequently recurring cold sores. My job is face-to-face sales, and when I get a cold sore, I try to stay home from work if I can. I've read a lot about suppression of genital herpes, but what about oral herpes? Can I take medicine every day to stop getting sores? Some studies show that daily therapy can reduce the frequency of cold sores too (Gilbert 2007). In fact, I often prescribe for this purpose. Both valacyclovir and famciclovir have approved doses for cold-sore treatment, but acyclovir doesn't and none have FDA approval for daily treatment. However, most clinicians will write these prescriptions. I recommend the genital-herpes suppression dose of any of the three medicines when used for daily therapy for cold sores. That dose should work well for most everyone.

My first really bad outbreak of genital herpes happened four months ago. I went on daily therapy immediately after finishing my first outbreak prescription. The original culture swab test from my sores was negative for herpes, and my antibody test was also negative for both types. My doctor wanted me to come back in four months for another antibody test, just to be sure she was right in her diagnosis. But now, the antibody test that I had done about a week ago was also negative. I'm completely confused! It's possible that your daily dosing of antiviral medicine has slowed the development of the antibody that's detected by blood tests. The purpose of the medicine is to reduce the amount of virus, right? If the medicine succeeds, that means there'll also be less virus around for the immune system to respond to, which it does through antibody production. I suggest that you stop taking medicine for a couple of months and then get tested again.

So we've talked about the various treatment options, comfort measures, and vaccines that are on the horizon. We'll now move on to talking about how to cope with having herpes. Let's be honest: this might be a real challenge, but herpes is manageable if you get your head on straight about the disease and really practice thinking differently about it.

Chapter 7

Telling Someone You Have Herpes

There are several people you might want to tell that you have herpes: family members; friends; and current, past, and prospective sex partners. You might feel motivated to tell them as a way to seek support, to unburden yourself of a secret, to notify someone who might also be infected, or as part of an attempt to clarify the source of your infection. Perhaps the most challenging discussion is the one you'll have with a potential sexual partner, so let's start with the hardest first.

TELLING POTENTIAL PARTNERS

Telling a potential partner that you have genital herpes is called "having the talk." It may not be easy, because many people have preconceived ideas about what it means to have genital herpes. In fact, it can be a downright tough one, and in this chapter we discuss reasons why you'd tell a potential partner, what to include in the discussion, at what point in the relationship to have "the talk," and even where to have it. When the proper time comes, you'll be prepared and eager to get started. Yeah, right! Well, at least you'll be well prepared.

Why Tell?

There are several reasons why you would disclose that you have genital herpes to a prospective partner before having sex:

It's what you would have wanted for yourself. I wonder whether you contracted herpes from someone who told you that he or she had it before the two of you had sex. Probably not. Most likely you got herpes from someone who didn't tell you ahead of time about the infection, either because the person didn't know he or she had it or because your partner felt that telling you about it was too difficult. You may not know for sure who gave you herpes. By telling a prospective partner that you have herpes and that he or she could contract it from you through sex, you're allowing the person to have a choice about whether or not to take that risk. You're acknowledging that this person would like to make a decision that belongs to him or her—a choice you, yourself, probably would've liked to have had before you were infected. Your prospective partner may accept or reject a sexual relationship with you based on this single thing about you, which can be a scary proposition because you're putting yourself on the line and risking rejection over a relatively minor health condition. But listen to the little voice inside your head for how to best handle this situation.

If you think talking about herpes is difficult *before* you become sexually intimate, picture having to admit to having herpes *after* you've transmitted it to a partner who's now sitting there looking at you, feeling hurt both physically and emotionally, and asking why you didn't disclose the facts earlier.

Sharing difficult information allows for greater intimacy and inspires trust. I'm sure you can think of other difficult information you've had to share in a successful relationship, right? Perhaps you had to declare bankruptcy, have an arrest record, got fired from an important job, or have a history of unsuccessful marriages or relationships. Those things may not involve genital sores, but they're still hard to talk about. Your partner will recognize that discussing herpes is a difficult subject to raise, and will most likely respect you for doing it and for giving him or her a choice about it. Your disclosing your herpes status will also set a precedent for your ability as a couple to bring up and discuss other difficult subjects. Once you've told your partner that you have herpes and put in place ways to manage it, you can start relaxing and enjoying the benefits of a close, intimate relationship, assured that you aren't keeping a secret that you know in your heart should be shared.

Telling partners about your herpes allows them to support you.
During outbreaks, when you might be having a difficult time emotionally with your herpes, it's great to have support from others. If you keep your herpes a secret, however, you deny your partner an opportunity to show you kindness and compassion during those tough times. And if you decide to withhold the knowledge about your infection, consider for a moment what you'll have to do during outbreaks. Will you become quiet and withdrawn, and reject sexual contact for no apparent reason? Your partner will wonder what's up and whether he or she's done something to upset you. Your partner might think the relationship is dying, which could lead to all kinds of confusion and mixed messages. The inability to communicate openly about herpes can lead to other unpleasant endings. You've certainly heard of "serial monogamy." I've had patients who practice something one might call "serial departure." They begin building an emotional attachment in a relationship, but when the relationship veers into the direction of sexuality, they become so nervous about disclosing their herpes status that they simply disappear, leaving their partners wondering what happened, and feeling confused and hurt, perhaps for years, about a relationship that ended for no discernable reason. This isn't fair to the uninfected, in-the-dark, "dumpee" partner, nor is it fair to the "dumper," who will probably never create a full and satisfying connection with anyone else using this counterproductive strategy. So think long and hard before adopting this method. On one hand, if you decide to risk telling your partner, you could either be rejected or accepted, so there are two possible outcomes: one good and one not so good. On the other hand, if you end the relationship to avoid having to tell, there's a 100 percent chance that the ending will be a bad one. By telling, you have at least half a chance, though my experience with patients indicates that your odds for continuing the relationship are far better than fifty-fifty.

If you tell an uninfected partner you have herpes, you're less likely to infect him or her. A study by Dr. Anna Wald at the University of Washington identified newly infected individuals (those with a positive swab test for HSV 2 and negative antibody test for HSV 2, proving first infection). She asked them a simple question: "Did you or did you not know that your partner had herpes when you started having sex with him or her?" If the answer was, "Yes, I knew my partner had herpes," the average time from beginning to have sex to the acquisition of herpes was 270 days. If the answer was, "No, I didn't know my partner had herpes," the average time to acquisition was 60 days (Wald et al. 2006a). There are likely several things going on to explain this very large difference in time to acquisition of infection. If your partner knows you have herpes, you'll feel comfortable saying things like, "It's probably not a good day to have sex. I feel a little tingling down there just now. How about if we make good use of our hands tonight!" But if you haven't disclosed your herpes status, you're more likely to take the risk of having genital sex because you wouldn't have a reasonable excuse not to. Or if you take suppressive therapy to reduce the risk of infecting a partner, you won't be tempted to do things like hide your medicine, fearing your partner might discover the bottle. Partners who know you're taking medicine can even help you remember to take your pills regularly. And if you want to use condoms to reduce the risk of transmission but haven't yet disclosed your herpes status, how might you respond to a request for alternative methods of birth control that don't provide the same protection as strict condom use? I'm sure you get the picture about all the benefits of having a partner "in the know" and on your side, rather than someone from whom you're trying to hide the truth.

One final thought: If an uninfected person is giving oral sex to an infected partner, with adequate lighting he or she can observe for any herpes symptoms that might be present on the genitals. This kind of mixes "business" with pleasure, but it's an effective risk-reduction strategy nonetheless.

You'll have an opportunity to challenge your own faulty beliefs. If you hold the belief that having genital herpes will result in no one ever again wanting to have sex with you, telling prospective partners allows you to test the validity of your belief. Most of my patients who've told prospective partners about their herpes are embraced, not rejected. But if you never tell anyone, you'll never get the chance to find out that your belief about automatically being rejected is wrong most of the time. True, a few people will say they don't want to take the risk, but many will be willing to do so if their relationship with you brings them other benefits and happiness.

It will open a dialogue about mutual testing for herpes and other STIs. It could be that your new partner is just waiting to have this discussion with you. Someone has to go first, right? It could just as easily be you as the other person. Your potential partner may feel incredibly relieved to have you bring this up, and be eternally grateful that you "opened the gates" of the herpes discussion.

Some people you tell about your herpes will react with surprise and say they're sure that they don't have it themselves. But prospective partners who believe they aren't infected with herpes will benefit from the clarity that their own lab tests can provide. You'll have done others a great service by encouraging them to get tested! It might take them a few days to start thinking about it like that, but in the long run you'll have allowed them to take control of something they needed to know about. Opening up about your condition also provides a great opportunity to give correct information to those who are uneducated about herpes (and that includes most of the population). And who's in a better position to start their education process than you, since you now have correct information from this book? In addition, if your partner is tested prior to when the two of you have sex, and you find out that he or she is already infected with HSV 2, you can have sex without further concern about herpes, because you can't pass the virus back and forth or trigger outbreaks in each other. Also, if your partner tests positive for herpes before you have sex rather than later on, when he or she notices symptoms, there will never be questions in your relationship about who gave what to whom and when.

It's probably a good thing to have all of these issues out in the open and on the table. When you tell someone you have genital herpes, it opens the door for talking about sexually transmitted infections in general. Sometimes, when we get so involved in thinking about herpes, we forget about the other STIs that can have much more serious health implications (see chapter 10). By talking about herpes, the conversation can naturally swing to discussing sexual health in general. Or you could do it in reverse: start talking about other STIs and then disclose your herpes.

You'll alleviate herpes concerns around a potential pregnancy. If children might be conceived in a relationship between someone who has herpes and someone who believes he or she isn't infected, herpes infection *must* be disclosed to protect the baby. The risk of neonatal herpes rises significantly when an infected partner (male or female) has sex with a pregnant woman who doesn't have herpes. If the infected person gives oral sex to the pregnant woman, the disclosure should include both genital and oral herpes status. We'll talk more about disclosing oral herpes status later in this chapter.

And finally, it's a legal matter. This part isn't much fun to think about, and I wish I didn't need to bring it up at all, but it really needs to be discussed in this age of dealing with our personal problems through the legal system. If you know that you have herpes and have sex with someone without telling him or her about it, and the person gets herpes, he or she can sue you under three different legal statutes: battery, misrepresentation, and negligence. The basis for all three causes of legal action is the assumption that disclosure must occur for the protection of uninfected partners and that, by honest disclosure, uninfected people have the opportunity to decide not to put themselves in the position of becoming infected. *Negligence* cases are based on a presumed "duty to act," to inform an uninfected partner that there's a possibility of "harm," which, in this case, is herpes infection. The legal concept of *battery* is based on intentional harm, that is, knowing that there's a risk of infecting someone else but failing to disclose that information. *Misrepresentation* is based on the presumption that false claims have been made, such as by making the statement, "I don't have any STIs," when you know that you do. Legal cases surrounding herpes aren't easy to prove, but very large sums of money have been awarded in some cases. As a herpes expert, I'm asked to review and comment on many herpes cases, and sometimes to testify in court. Although the legal technicalities escape me most of the time, the negative feelings, the anxiety and sadness, of these situations do not. Who'd ever want to go through such hassles, anyway? It's just way easier to tell the truth about herpes.

Let's summarize all of the reasons for disclosing your herpes status before having sex with someone who doesn't know. Reviewing this list each time you plan to have "the talk" will clarify for you why you're about to put yourself through this challenging interaction.

Review of Reasons to Tell

- It's what you would have wanted for yourself. Your potential partners will wish to decide for themselves whether to risk getting herpes.

- Sharing difficult information in a relationship inspires trust and intimacy.

- Knowing that you have herpes gives your partner the opportunity to be supportive of you when you need it.

- When you tell and your partner knows, the risk of transmitting herpes to him or her goes down.

- You'll have a chance to challenge any erroneous beliefs you have about herpes and potentially getting rejected.

- Telling opens up a discussion about herpes testing of your partner as well as other STI testing.

- A future pregnancy will be safer if herpes is known to be involved.

- If you don't disclose that you have herpes and you transmit it, you could be sued and go through months or years of legal misery, with all of its potentially devastating financial consequences.

Whom Do You Tell and How Soon?

It's probably not a good strategy to pull up a bar stool next to someone you've just met and say something like, "Hi, my name's Linda, and I have genital herpes." Take your time and be selective about whom you tell. You may find that having herpes changes the nature of your sexual relationships. The amount of time that passes in a relationship before people have sex has gotten shorter over the years, but having herpes often extends the time frame. There are other things you'll probably wait to disclose about yourself until you get to know someone better, but disclosing herpes is a little different because it has to do with the timing of first sexual encounters. You'll need to figure out the timing of "the talk" so that it happens somewhere between "hello" and before penetration. By the way, you don't have to tell partners before you have *any* sexual contact—just the kind that might transmit infection to a partner. For some couples, sex begins in a matter of days; for others, months; and for others, it'll be the day they get married. How to find the best time to disclose varies greatly from couple to couple, but here are a few considerations for knowing if you're even telling the right person.

Should You Tell This Person?

How well do you know this person? Has the person disclosed difficult or private things to you—perhaps about his or her background, family, or life before meeting you—that indicates the person can appreciate and handle vulnerability? Have you talked about what this person values, what issues matter to him or her, and what guides the way the person moves through his or her life? Do you get the sense that this person can put things into a reasonable perspective? Has this person ever discussed characteristics or habits about himself or herself that he or she would like to change, or does this person seem to think that he or she is just about perfect?

How much do you trust this person with something very personal? How certain do you feel that this person will respect your privacy regarding the news about herpes? The last thing you want is to read a post to someone's social-networking Web page about your genital herpes or to experience a similar public revealing! You want to be clear that your partner respects the importance of privacy about this disclosure. Where does this person fit into your circle of friends? Do you feel that, in spite of this person's close relationships with others in your circle, he or she can keep this information private? Once you disclose your herpes status, there's some risk of your being "outed" about your herpes; this may be the one real downside of disclosure, but it could be a really big one.

Is this person open to learning new things? Does this person have his or her mind made up about most things already, or is he or she open to new ideas and learning opportunities? In most cases, people who believe they're uninfected but haven't actually been tested would benefit from a lab test to confirm or deny this belief. But the person who's dead sure about most things—you know, the "I've made up my mind, don't confuse me with the facts" type—probably wouldn't agree to testing and would be reluctant to learn more about genital herpes anyway. Imagine how the scenario would look if you asked someone like that to get tested for herpes; how might the response go?

Is It Time to Tell?

It's best to wait until you know that a relationship is really going somewhere before you raise the issue of herpes. If there's no emotional bond between the two of you, your partner is less likely to take the risk of getting herpes. That certainly makes sense anyway, right? It helps if there's been some investment in the relationship that might make someone willing to take the risk of getting genital herpes.

You might be the kind of person who approaches disclosure differently. Perhaps you want to get "the talk" out of the way, so you tell prospective partners very early on in the relationship. Some people believe that it's wrong to "lead people on" too far into the relationship without telling them about their herpes, because somehow that means they've wasted someone else's time. But I disagree with that concept. No one puts all their cards on the table right away about all their personal stuff. We each hold back things for a while until trust is built. Why is herpes any different? Sometimes you might have "the talk" early on, as a way of testing someone's intentions or sincerity, but I wonder if that comes more from feelings of self-doubt than from a need to be totally honest early on. For some people, it's almost as if they're saying in their heads, "Okay, I know you'll probably reject me, so I'm just going to blurt it out, have it over with, and move on; so why not just do it now?" But that's not operating from a position of strength and reason. It's coming from a defensive position, and such fear-based people are sometimes rejected, because the scene plays out according to their own self-fulfilling prophecies.

There's no perfect time to bring up the subject of having herpes, but some opportunities may present themselves that can help you. Once you know that it's almost time to have "the talk," start looking for good openings.

Opportunities for Telling

Herpes Medicine TV Ads: How lucky you are if there happens to be a herpes medicine commercial airing on TV when you want to share the news! They're on pretty frequently these days, so it could happen! You could say something like: *"Hey, have you noticed that those commercials are on quite a bit now? I think it's great that these issues are being brought right out into the open these days, don't you?"*

Herpes Jokes: Have you ever been at a gathering where someone told a herpes joke? Maybe before you got herpes, it wasn't a big deal, or maybe, even then, you objected to the insensitivity. But now you can use those jokes as an opening to talk about your own disease: *"Did you hear that herpes joke at the party tonight? It bothered me a little, and I almost said something about it at the time and now kind of wish I had, but how did you feel about it?"*

The STI Version: At some point prior to having sex that might expose your partner to herpes, it's important to talk about sexually transmitted infections in general, such as when you were each last tested for STIs, which ones were included, and so on. Again, it doesn't have to be *any* sexual contact; there are lots of fun sexual things you can do that don't present a risk, and in fact, that might not be a bad thing at all. You'll get more of a feel (so to speak) for your overall attraction to this person and his or her attraction to you! So you could say something like: *"Is it just me, or is the temperature in this room getting hotter? Whew! If we're going to have more sex in the near future, and I'd say that's pretty likely, what would you think about our making appointments to get tested for all those STIs out there? I really think that's best for both of us, don't you? And before we do that, I'd like to tell you a little (more) about my sexual history, and maybe you'd like to share something (more) about yours too."*

The "We're Moving Ahead" Version: This is a very common opportunity that many people take. As things in the relationship warm up emotionally and heat up sexually, it becomes the appropriate thing to discuss: *"Well, it seems to me that we're moving into a more physical relationship than we've had up until now, and if you agree, there's something I'd like to share with you."*

Leaving This Book on the Coffee Table: Do you find it difficult to get the first words out of your mouth? An alternative option would be to leave this book on the coffee table when you feel that things are moving in the direction of sex. It's pretty unlikely it'll go unnoticed, don't you think? That way, your partner will probably ask you why it's there, and you can begin to talk about herpes: *"So, I see you looking at my book there. Interesting title, don't you think? Kind of makes you wonder what's inside. The truth is, I put that book out tonight so we could talk about something that's personally important to me. Is this a good time?"*

The "You May Be Wondering Why We Haven't Had Sex Yet" Version: You've been going out for about six months, and although you don't disapprove of sex before marriage on religious or moral grounds, you've still not consummated the relationship, and the issue is in the room like the proverbial unacknowledged elephant. You're scared, really scared. You've been looking for just the right moment, nothing ever seems to click, and you've been tempted on numerous occasions to just skip the talk and do the deed, but something always holds you back. Your partner is clearly confused: Is it you, is it him or her, do you dislike sex, have you suffered sexual trauma at some point, do you have other "issues"? It's time to tell; you know it is, and you can do this! *"I'm sure you've been wondering for weeks why I've been postponing having sex with you. You've been patient and very dear, and I want to be clear that this isn't so much about you. I'm really attracted to you, and I know you're attracted to me, so that's all terrific. But there's something I haven't yet shared with you, and it's time I did, so here goes."*

The Style of "the Talk"

How you talk about something sets the stage for how it's heard. Sometimes the message itself is overshadowed by the way in which the listener hears it. Take herpes, for example. If, while you're shaking and tearful, you say to a potential partner, "I have the most awful thing to tell you, and I'm sure that when I'm done, you'll run the other way," he or she probably will. If, on the other hand, you phrase things differently, you may get a much better response. Keep the introduction to the topic simple. Don't go on and on. Consider these two options:

Scenario A: *"Before we have sex, there's something very personal I'd like to share with you. I've had genital herpes for about four years now, and it's not a big deal for me, but I feel it's fair to let you know up front."*

Scenario B: *"Before we have sex, there's something very private that I need to say to you, and if you tell anyone else, I'll be totally mortified. It's pretty devastating, and you aren't going to like it one bit, but I can't help it. I'll totally understand if you want to leave right now and run the other way. Other people have, and it's never a surprise when it happens. I mean, what else can I expect? A real jerk did this to me, and I'll never do it to someone else, but the jerk did to me, so here I am, putting myself on the line. Are you ready? Buckle your seat belt; have I got news for you!"*

Which scenario do you think plays better, A or B? Which will get the best results? Of course, it's A, but it's worth thinking for a minute about how you felt in your gut when you read B. That's how it's heard if you present herpes in that way to someone else.

The Setting

Choose the best answer to complete the following sentence:
The best time and place to tell a partner that you have herpes is…

A. In your favorite bar at happy hour.

B. In bed as one of you is slipping on a condom.

C. On your patio having some dessert.

I know—you probably said, "Duh!" when you read my questions. I've got to start making these harder. But yes, of course, answer C is the best. Discussions like this are better held in a private, quiet place and not just prior to having herpes-risk sex. The location should allow for an intimate and detailed discussion, and although tears aren't ideal, they sometimes come anyway.

Contents of "the Talk"

Though partners should have the opportunity to ask questions, they may not have a clue what to ask, so you might need to somewhat lead the conversation by giving some information. Here are the basics that should be included in any discussion of herpes:

Herpes is a sexually transmitted infection. *"You won't get it from kissing or touching me, using my toilet, or sleeping in my bed. It requires sex to get it."*

One out of every five people over the age of eighteen in the United States has genital herpes, and of those, 90 percent don't even know they have it. *"Unless you've been tested, there's a chance you're infected but just don't know it. There's no way to know for sure except a lab test. I know where to get one if you're interested. And even if you've had STI testing in the past, most doctors and STI clinics don't include testing for herpes, but you could call and check on that."*

I'm on a daily medicine (if you really are) that reduces the risk of infecting you by a lot. *"If we use condoms, the risk goes down even more. I'm aware of the symptoms that happen before I get an outbreak, so we should avoid sex during those times of extra risk. But nothing is perfect for protecting you. There's still a small chance I could give you herpes in spite of all our best efforts."* (Note: Depending upon your partner's gender, cite the numbers we talked about in chapter 3 to provide an idea of how common transmission is and isn't.)

You don't have to decide right now whether to have sex with me. *"In fact, I'd really prefer that you to take some time to think about all this so that you're absolutely clear about your decision. I told you this now so that you could make an informed decision, and that doesn't come instantly. If you're interested, I have a book you can borrow to learn more about herpes. If you still want to be intimate, we can do other perfectly safe sexual stuff instead of intercourse right now, or we could just snuggle, but I really want you to take your time."*

This is very personal for me. *"It's not something I tell everyone, because there's just no need to tell everyone, and I hope you'll respect my privacy by not sharing this with other people. Telling your doctor would be okay if you want to get tested or discuss this with a professional, but not friends or family, please. Let's just keep this between you and me. Can you understand why I feel this way? Are you okay with that?"*

Whatever you decide about this, I really like you. *"I understand that this isn't easy—for either of us. Most people feel comfortable living with the small risk of getting herpes, but others don't."*

Keep the first discussion relatively brief, unless your partner asks lots of questions. And be prepared for your partner to take the time you've offered him or her to think about it. Your partner would certainly be smart to do that.

Possible Responses

Instant Acceptance: If your partner says, "I don't need to think about this for even five minutes. You're the hottest thing in my life, and nothing could stop me from being with you!" that's all very nice—maybe. Your expectation was that your partner would consider the information and make an informed decision, because when hormones override reason, regrets could follow. Your partner doesn't necessarily have to leave your presence to think about it, but a day of pondering would only make everyone feel clearer about the choices at hand. If your partner says something sweet like, "I love you no matter what you have; don't you know that?" it becomes even more tempting to just go ahead and have sex, but try to still give things a little time. Everyone's body parts will still be around and functioning in a few hours, or a day or two.

Instant Rejection: Let's say the response is, *"Herpes!* Are you kidding? I thought you were a clean person! There's no way I'm taking a risk like that; I have a whole life ahead of me!" That, of course, is much harder to take. On one hand, however, you'd know that you're dealing with someone who isn't showing compassion or concern about you, and in the long run, he or she might just not have been the best partner for you anyway. Or maybe the person just has incorrect information about herpes, along with a whole set of unreasonable fears, and he or she will mellow out after a few days of thinking about it. But in the short run, hearing such words is painful, and they come from a place of ignorance about herpes. You may need to remind yourself repeatedly that you're a person with much to offer and that this is a reaction that happens infrequently. There's more to learn about how to deal with rejection in chapter 8. Suffice it to say, the person is rejecting the herpes, not you.

Surprise: Perhaps your partner will look at you with astonishment and say something like, "Wow, I don't know anything about herpes, and I don't know what to say to you now." That's really a fairly common response, and it's an ideal opening to do some educating. You can say, *"That's okay; lots of people don't know much about herpes, but I've got some really good things for you to read and a video* (see chapter 11) *you can watch if you'd like. For now, would you like me to tell you a little more about it?"* Try to keep your message simple and clear, and as unemotional as possible. You don't have to be a robot, but crying may give the message that herpes is definitely something to be very sad about, and that's probably not the message you want to give.

Long-Term Indecision: You told your prospective partner three months ago, and you've discussed herpes together several times since then. The person has read this book and even gone in for a blood antibody test showing that he or she doesn't have herpes. Foreplay has been great and fun, but it never goes beyond that. You're taking your medicine regularly, and you've been checking for symptoms and haven't noticed any. The condoms are in your drawer, just waiting for their moment in the sun (or in the dark), but your partner just can't decide what to do. Your partner is, in a word, stuck. "You're great," the person says, everything he or she could've hoped for in a life partner, but the idea of herpes is bothersome. Your partner is "so into you," except for *that*. With each week that passes, you feel just a little less desirable, a little "one down," somehow worth a little less than the person who doesn't have herpes. You wonder if this is how it's always going to be, with your partners remaining undecided about whether you would be an acceptable sex partner.

Stop right there! You're in a very bad situation, and despite the fact that I'd like to tell you otherwise, it'll probably just stay that way or get worse. Over the years, I've counseled many couples in this situation, and I've rarely seen one like this turn out well. After months of pondering, you begin to get slightly depressed and doubt your overall desirability as a partner. The uninfected person doesn't leave but doesn't consummate the relationship either. And, if he or she does have intercourse, there's lots of hand and genital washing immediately after sex, and the messages that accompany those behaviors are not cheery. This can become a distinctly downward spiral. If you're in this situation, I reluctantly encourage you to step back and step out. The odds are very high that this just isn't a good match for you. The mixed messages you're getting from this situation can cause you long-term difficulties. Believe it or not, there'll be others who'll accept you as you are, but you'll never find them while you're stuck in this quagmire. Moving on will probably be difficult, but it's the best thing for both of you under the circumstances. I wish I could suggest otherwise.

TELLING OTHERS

You may not want to tell lots of people that you have genital herpes, but telling at least one person is important. Some people find that this is a big secret to carry around all by themselves. When you do share this information, you'll probably find that there are others in your situation. Others you might want to tell are your current or past sex partners, family, or friends. Let's begin with telling your current partner, which can get tricky because you might be worried that he or she will think that you've been cheating. There are many possible scenarios in this situation.

Telling a Current Partner

You've been married and monogamous for nine years, and you've never had any symptoms of genital herpes. Three days ago, however, you woke up with a group of blisters on your buttocks that hurt and itched. You went to an urgent-care clinic, where they swabbed the blisters and called you back this morning to tell you that the swab was positive for herpes simplex virus. You're shocked, angry and completely confused. How could this happen to you? You've had other sex partners in your life, but that was before you got married! You're thinking that if you were infected years prior, you would've known, right? You're thinking that your spouse surely cheated and gave you herpes. You start searching the yellow pages for the meanest divorce lawyer you can find.

But hold on! It's very important to remember that there are several possible scenarios here. One is that you really have had genital herpes for years and didn't know it. Another possibility is that your partner has been infected for years and either did or didn't know about it. A third possibility is that you have genital HSV 1 from receiving oral sex from your partner; there was no typing on the swab test result, so you need to clear up that question right away. And, yes, the final possibility is that you or your partner had sex with another person, and an "open relationship" wasn't part of your agreement. This last one is obviously the most difficult and unpleasant scenario, but it's the one most people jump to first, and that's often a big mistake. It would be unfair (and embarrassing) to accuse your partner of having been unfaithful if you were the only one who turned out to be infected and your partner were the one at risk of getting infected from you!

The Position of Confusion

Since there are several possible explanations for your infection, it's best to take the "position of confusion" when you talk with your partner. When you bring up the subject, it's good if it goes something like this: *"I've just talked to the urgent-care clinic about those blisters on my hip, and the news is that I have genital herpes. This is really confusing to me, because I've never noticed those symptoms before. The physician assistant who gave me the results told me I could've had this for years without knowing it, that you could've had it for years without knowing it and just passed it to me, or that it could be from your giving me oral sex, so it could be the cold-sore virus. I'll find out about that for sure in a few days. I feel pretty confident that you haven't had any other partners, and I know I haven't, so I guess that leaves us with some unanswered questions. Can we try to sort this out together?"*

You get the idea. There's no blaming, no plates flying through the air, and no accusations being tossed around. There's only confusion, and the confusion is very real. If some of these possibilities are not true for you (for example, you've never had another sex partner, or you don't receive oral sex), then you have to shape the message to fit your own situation, of course. But if you and your partner have had sex with other people in your lifetimes and you practice oral sex, then all of those other scenarios are still on the table. Further testing of your swab sample and antibody testing of your spouse will provide you with more information about what's happened here.

Are you afraid that your partner will think that you've been unfaithful, so you're frightened about raising the issue? That's a very common fear, but you know in your heart what's true about your own fidelity, right? If you've been monogamous, then you must simply deal with the circumstances as they are. If you want to wait until typing of the virus is back before bringing this up, that's okay too. But at some point, you'll want to discuss this issue with your spouse.

Scenarios with Your Long-Term Partner or Spouse

- If your swab test is positive for HSV 2, your blood antibody test is positive for HSV 2, both of you've had other partners, and your partner's blood antibody test is also positive, you'll never know where the virus came from. You could've given it to your partner, your partner could've given it to you, or someone in the past could've given it to either of you. It's just there and need not be a significant factor in your relationship.

- If your swab test is positive for HSV 2, your antibody test is positive for HSV 2, and your partner is antibody negative for type 2, then you've likely had herpes for years and didn't know it, and you could potentially infect your partner at some point in the future.

- If your swab test is positive for HSV 2, your blood antibody test is negative for HSV 2, and your spouse's blood antibody test is positive for HSV 2, then your partner probably recently infected you. If your partner has had sex with other people prior to you, then your spouse could've had herpes for years and just didn't know it. Or your partner could've been infected in the past several months and has already made antibody. There is simply no way to know. But now that you're both infected, herpes transmission is not a worry in your sex life.

- If your swab test is positive for HSV 1, your antibody test is positive for HSV 1, and your spouse is also antibody positive for HSV 1, then you've both been infected with HSV 1 for some time. In this case, too, transmission is no longer a worry in your sex life.

- If your swab test is positive for HSV 2, your antibody test is negative for HSV 2, and your partner's antibody test is also negative for HSV 2, the situation becomes a bit more confusing. One explanation is that your partner recently acquired HSV 2 from someone else, and though not enough time has passed to make antibody, he or she was infectious and just now infected you. In this case, a repeat antibody testing of your partner will help clarify the situation. However, if you and your partner become antibody positive at the same time and both of you deny having had another partner, one of you may not be telling the whole story. Another possibility is that the antibody test has failed to detect existing antibody in you or your partner. This is more likely to happen with HSV 1 than 2.

- If your swab test is positive for HSV 1 and your antibody test is negative for HSV 1, and your partner gets cold sores and also gives you oral sex, then it's likely that your partner infected you with genital HSV 1, even if a cold sore wasn't present when he or she gave you oral sex.

If you're afraid that your partner will accuse you of infidelity, try thinking about this another way. Let's say that you've been monogamous but decide against disclosing your recent diagnosis out of fear of recrimination and accusations. But a year down the road, your partner has a herpes outbreak that gets accurately diagnosed. Where will your partner point the finger? At you. And you'll have known that you've had herpes all that time but kept it a secret. What will your partner think about that? Why the secrecy? What were you hiding all that time? It's far better to face the music and deal with the fallout right away.

Telling Previous Partners

Often people ask, "Do I have to let my past sexual partners know about this, and if yes, how far back do I have to go to make those notifications?" There's no perfect answer here. If you feel you want to make previous partners aware that you have herpes so that they can be tested (either because you think they infected you or you may have infected them), that's fine. But it's unclear whether you really have to do that. Again, this will depend upon the nature of your relationship with past partners and how things ended.

Telling Family Members

Whether you tell any family members surely depends upon the relationship you have with them. For some of you, your mom, dad, or both will be your first confidants, but for others, they would be the absolute last to tell, if at all. If you decide to tell your folks, remember that, for most parents, loving and supporting you is a top priority. So even though this is about you and sex, which might be awkward for you to talk about, Mom or Dad will soon move past that aspect and focus on how you're coping with having herpes rather than how you got it. Sometimes telling close siblings is easier, because they're closer to your age, but if you aren't close to any of your siblings, it may not be a good idea to disclose it to them.

Telling Friends

For most of you, your closest friend will be the first person you'll tell. There's no sexual history, no judgment, and no fear of being accused of cheating. Besides, it's safe, easy, and important to share this information with someone you trust. Friends sometimes respond that they, too, have herpes. But will they keep your diagnosis to themselves? If confidentiality matters, then make that clear. As with partners, be aware when you share. This is private news, and it would be nice for you to be able to pick and choose who knows. You can also reassure your friend that herpes is not transmitted by using toilet seats or through casual, nonsexual contact.

Employers and Coworkers

Remember our discussion of how herpes is a sexually transmitted infection and isn't passed to others by using toilet seats and touching doorknobs? If you aren't having sex with your coworkers, they don't need to know that you have herpes.

Health Care Providers

Your ob-gyn diagnosed your genital herpes; do you have to share that information with your family-practice provider? How about your eye doctor? When your dentist gives you the form to fill out that lists your medicines, do you have to tell him or her about the acyclovir you're taking? That's all optional. However, the best health care is possible when your clinician is aware of all your health issues, but not everything is relevant to every visit. And luckily, there are no interactions between herpes medicines and other drugs. Think about how, or if, your herpes impacts the care you're receiving or the procedures that are happening, and make your decisions appropriately. For example, if you're having a facial plastic-surgery procedure, oral herpes should be disclosed. If you're having back surgery, it would be good to be on suppressive therapy to avoid sparking an outbreak. And if you're having a baby, you know you must tell your OB provider. You get the picture. However, for example, if you're having your teeth cleaned, you don't need to share with your dentist that you have genital herpes.

WHAT IF YOU HAD SEX BUT DIDN'T TELL FIRST?

If you went ahead and had sex without disclosing your herpes status, you probably did it for one of three reasons:

- You were afraid of being rejected.

- You misjudged the nature of the relationship.

- You believed you weren't infectious at the time.

The first is probably the most common reason people don't tell a partner: the fear that a partner would think less of you and not want to continue the relationship. But the problem with doing that is trading one problem for another: the potential loss of a partner's trust. In the big picture, however, that's not an equal trade-off, is it? At some point, you'll need to tell your partner that you have herpes, either because it becomes too large of a secret to carry or because you'll have infected your partner and the matter will have become quite evident. But then your partner will begin to think, if not say, "What else have you not told me?" or in other words, "What else have you lied to me about?" You partner may understand your reluctance, but he or she still won't like it. Trust is so important in a relationship. It takes a long time to build but moments to lose. If you haven't told your sex partner yet, now is the time. Explain your fears, ask your partner to forgive you for this error, promise to be more open with difficult issues in the future, and hope that he or she is willing to move on despite your mistake. But don't wait until next week; tell your partner now.

The second possibility, that of misjudging the nature of the relationship, usually happens when you think you're having a casual sexual encounter and don't feel the need to share your most personal secrets with someone with whom you might not have sex again. However, the sex turns out to have been wonderful, you feel a different level of connection, and you want to spend more time with that person. Now you've backed yourself into a small corner. A subject that you thought you wouldn't have to broach is now front and center. The solution's the same as for the first scenario. Tell your partner as soon as possible, explain what you were thinking, ask for forgiveness, and hope that he or she can let this pass and continue to build the relationship with you.

What if you don't tell a casual sexual partner that you have herpes, the relationship doesn't go anywhere, and you feel that this is okay as a regular practice and won't be persuaded otherwise. You think the odds are so low that it isn't worth the social stigma to tell. This is actually common and, in some ways, understandable. From a scientific point of view, the person you want to have sex with long term and the person you want to have sex with just for tonight are equally vulnerable with each sexual encounter, right? In one situation, the regular partner may get to find out, but in the case of the casual partner, he or she doesn't get to find out. Is it really about the nature of the relationship or the possibility of transmission? Does the person you love have more of a right to know that he or she is at risk of getting herpes than the person you have sex with casually? Does the fact that your casual partner agrees to have casual sex with you somehow make him or her less entitled to the information necessary to protect himself or herself from herpes? Do you think that if someone agrees to have casual sex with you that all bets are off, that this person has inherently agreed to take certain risks? Do you think it's okay to play Follow the Leader with a bad leader? I really don't claim to have the perfect answer, and certainly, the couple who has unprotected casual sex without benefit of condoms is taking some risk. But put yourself in the place of your partner: would you have wanted to know that there was a risk of getting herpes, a condition that you would have for the remainder of your life, before you had sex? What guides you in decisions like these? These questions may not drive you to tell casual partners, but I hope they provide you with food for thought.

The third situation is often caused by the advice of medical professionals. You were told that you couldn't transmit herpes when you don't have an outbreak, when you use condoms, or when you're on suppressive medication. Except now you know, after reading this book, that those statements are false and that there's always a small possibility that you can infect a partner, even if you're doing all the right things to reduce the risk. The task ahead is to now tell your partner that you have herpes but previously had wrong information about how it's transmitted.

In all of these situations, recommend that your partner seek antibody testing, and I recommend that you offer to pay for his or her testing.

You can expect your partner to be disconcerted about the situation, and in the next chapter we'll talk about the psychological and emotional impacts of having genital herpes in the event that you've infected your partner.

QUESTIONS AND ANSWERS ABOUT TELLING OTHERS YOU HAVE HERPES

I've been married for ten years, and this week, I went in to see my doctor because I keep getting these painful boils on my butt. He diagnosed me as having HSV 2 from a swab test of the boil! I can't believe it! I'm so afraid to tell my husband, because he'll think I've been cheating on him and he'll be so mad that he'll leave me. I've never had sex with anyone else since we've been married. What should I do? You know you haven't had sex with anyone else. You should tell your husband about this. Either of you could've been infected for years before you met, if you've had other sex partners in your lifetime. If you've never had sex with anyone else, then you know that he has at some time in his life. If you know that he had other partners before you, he could've had herpes for years before he met you. A strong marriage can handle this news, because a strong marriage has trust. If your marriage isn't the greatest, then it may not survive this. But if your husband doesn't believe you, in spite of things like this to read or information from your clinician, then you're in far more trouble than having herpes. What is, is. You've just found out what is, and it isn't about your having done anything shameful. If you fear your husband, be careful here. If there's a chance that he could hurt you, you need to take care of yourself. But remember, if you don't tell him and he finds out later, he'll wonder why you kept this from him, and saying that you were afraid may not be enough to satisfy his anger.

I have genital herpes, and I'd rather be alone for the rest of my life than risk being rejected by someone I tell. It's that simple. That's a pretty strong response but one I've heard from other people, most often in the first few months of being infected. Perhaps it boils down to exploring what rejection means to you. Does it mean that you're worthless? Does it mean that you have so little meaning that you can be tossed out for something as simple as an occasional genital sore? Usually, when people absolutely refuse to take the risk of being rejected, it has to do with low self-esteem and lack of self-acceptance. I hope you'll read the next chapter, which shares some ways to debate these negative and lonely thoughts. You can stand being rejected; you can live through that. It won't be fun, but you can stand it, and depending on how you put it, I think you'll be accepted far more often than rejected. Get yourself an imaginary scale: Put being alone for the rest of your life on one side and being rejected by someone on the other. Now what do you see? Is the balance shifting? Can you see how a lifetime alone might not be worth a rejection? I hope so.

I usually tell new partners that I have herpes on the very first date. Otherwise, they'll just be bummed that they wasted time on me when I do tell them. I'm just being very up-front and honest, and honesty is always the best policy, right? And if they reject me, fine; *they weren't worth the trouble anyway.* So, are you this honest about all aspects of your being or just herpes?

You see, I think some things are best kept to yourself until you know someone more intimately. Can you think of other things that you keep to yourself until later in the relationship? And why do you do that? Do you know? Are you waiting to share personal things until you know and trust your partner more? There's an element of protection that all of us employ when meeting new people. There are psychotic people on the street who tell you everything, but that really isn't healthy. Most of us measure out our personal information as we feel it's warranted, based on the level of the relationship. The same is true of herpes. When you build something first, some level of trust and interest, the person you tell has something to grasp onto, a reason to take a risk. Also, I sense some anger in your question. Do you think you could be just *daring* the person to reject you, to confirm something that you think you already know about him or her; or more, something you think about yourself? Think about it just a bit.

So now you know how to treat herpes and how to tell people that you have it, but there's still this unpleasant feeling down deep. In the next chapter, let's talk about how to think differently about herpes.

Chapter 8

Psychological Response to Genital Herpes: Getting Your Head on Straight

In a telephone survey conducted by the American Social Health Association in 2004 (Gilbert et al. 2005), 96 percent of randomly chosen respondents said they'd find a diagnosis of HIV infection "very traumatic." Close behind, 68 percent said that a diagnosis of genital herpes would also be "very traumatic." For a bit of perspective, 54 percent found breaking up with a significant other "very traumatic," and 51 percent said the same about getting fired from their jobs. In this survey, two thirds of those interviewed viewed genital herpes as equally upsetting to breaking up with a partner and losing a job. But wait just a minute. Is there anything you've read so far in this book that suggests that genital herpes is a terrible thing—medically speaking? No, there isn't. But as you can see from the survey results, a genital herpes diagnosis is never just a medical thing. It's an emotional, psychological, and relationship issue. Again, herpes is a condition that's socially stigmatized way out of proportion to its medical implications.

And although you may have had a difficult first outbreak, you now know that the physical symptoms of future herpes outbreaks can be easily managed with medication. So what's the big deal about genital herpes? Well, it's how you *feel* about herpes that makes it a big deal.

So, let's talk a bit about the common emotional reactions you may experience when you get diagnosed with genital herpes. But please understand, it's not that you're *supposed* to have these feelings. If you don't, that's fine, but if you do, you're in good company with many others who feel the same way.

EARLY EMOTIONAL RESPONSES

People seem to go through two separate periods in their reactions to having herpes. The first obviously comes right away; it starts as you sit in your clinician's office and hear the words, "I think you may have herpes," and continues until you get your test results that confirm those suspicions. When the news first hits, your thinking may be scattered, so it's hard to sit there, listen, and learn. Your own thoughts are racing: how long have I had this, who gave it to me, and what will I do now? You might have the best-informed, most compassionate clinician there is, but your inability to process anything but your emotions interferes with your ability to absorb what you're being told about herpes. You may have run out to a bookstore immediately and found this book, but you're still flipping randomly through the pages, trying to gather your thoughts. All of this, however, is perfectly normal and expected. Let's talk specifically about some of the reactions you may have had early on, right after you got the news.

Shock and Surprise

When you were first diagnosed, you were probably shocked that something like this could ever happen to you and to discover that you now have a lifelong sexually transmitted infection. These realities may have caused you to cry and ask, "Why me?" especially since you thought you were careful and never saw it coming. It's completely okay to feel shock, surprise, and a sense of disbelief when you're diagnosed with herpes. Of course, if you knew that your partner had herpes beforehand and you understood the risk of getting infected, you're probably not as surprised. But even in that situation, you may have held the belief that you'd be the one to "dodge the bullet."

Anger

Your anger could've been directed at a number of people, but the first may have been your partner: "How could you do this to me?" "How dare you give me genital herpes?" "You must've been cheating on me!" But the cold and simple reality is that you could've been the one who had herpes first. Or, if you really do have a new infection, your partner may not have known about being infected; remember that about 90 percent of those who have herpes don't know it (Leone et al. 2004). It's normal to wonder if your partner was unfaithful, particularly if you've been together for a long time, but remember that monogamous couples can be together for years before transmission occurs. I've seen this many times in my practice, so if you're skeptical about this possibility, it really does happen. Playing the 'blame game" won't change the fact that you have herpes; so what's the point in doing it? You may never be able to sort out who gave what to whom. You can either have herpes plus a contentious relationship with your partner over this issue, or you can simply have herpes. It's your choice.

You might be angry with your clinician. You'd always been diligent about asking for regular STI testing before entering a new sexual relationship, and now you find out that herpes screening was never included. "How could that be?" you ask. "How could I not have been tested for the most common STI in America when I specifically asked for a full STI screen?" Or it could be that your herpes diagnostic visit was less than ideal. Perhaps your clinician didn't provide much information or education, or failed to address your emotional needs. Maybe you feel that you were rushed in and out of the appointment, or that your concerns were minimized. Perhaps the clinical staff even made you feel ashamed or embarrassed about getting herpes. Maybe a clinician had told your sex partner that herpes could be transmitted only during an outbreak, so you found out the hard way that this isn't true.

Your anger could be directed at society for having such a negative view of STIs and stigmatizing a common infection. But the person at whom you're most angry may be you. Either recently or long ago, you put yourself in a position to be infected with genital herpes: you didn't have every sex partner tested for STIs before having sex, didn't use condoms with every encounter, had a casual encounter you regretted, or weren't faithful to your regular partner and thus contracted herpes.

Your sexual behavior was, in your view, less than perfect, so now you're beating yourself up emotionally for it.

Sometimes people say to me, "I have a *right* to be angry about contracting herpes: I never had a choice!" or "I have a *right* to be angry: my partner cheated on me and gave me herpes!" Maybe you really do have a right to be angry, and for some amount of time, and to some degree, you will be. But after a while you'll need to decide whether or not your anger is helping you in some way or if it's just making you unhappy. How, you ask, can anger help? If your partner has a history of having sex with other people, but you've both agreed to monogamy, your anger may propel you out of an unhealthy relationship, which might be a good thing. But if you're mad at the person who gave you herpes and they didn't even know they had it, or if you're harboring hostile feelings toward someone who simply didn't tell you he or she was infected for one of several reasons that made sense to him or her at the time, you'll need to ask yourself how long you want to keep that up. If you redirect the energy you're using to be angry into moving forward, I believe you'll be far better off in the long run.

Guilt

Guilt is a form of anger at yourself that involves a troubled conscience about something you've done that creates a conflict between how you perceive right and wrong, and your actions. Having sex with someone other than your regular partner, and getting herpes in the process, is a situation that often elicits guilty feelings. Not only have you violated your promise to be monogamous, but now you also have an infection that can't be cured and that can be passed to your partner through one of life's most intimate expressions of love and affection. The resulting guilt can immobilize you and cause great sadness.

Another emotion you might feel is regret. Regret is similar to guilt or remorse but without the bothered conscience: you feel bad for a behavior and vow to try to avoid making a similar error again in the future. Regret may be more useful than guilt, because it lets you move yourself into areas where you can act differently, whereas guilt often just weighs you down with negative feelings about yourself and sometimes makes you unable to move ahead and do better.

Confusion

If you're like most people diagnosed with genital herpes, you knew very little about the disease. Oh sure, you may have heard about it in a high-school health class. Maybe you even have a friend with herpes, but you never paid any serious attention to this particular infection. But now, you're scrambling to learn all you can in a short period of time. However, depending upon how much information you received from your clinician when you were diagnosed, you may find yourself struggling to set this all straight in your head. HSV 1, HSV 2, mouths, genitals, shedding, blood tests, swab tests, old infection, new infection, suppression, outbreak treatment—no wonder you're confused! And believe me, too many clinicians are just as confused as you are about the details of genital herpes. Unless you have the time and interest to focus on this topic for a while, it'll be difficult to keep things straight.

You can clear up a lot of confusion through self-education and by asking your clinician a few questions about how your diagnosis was made. Get as much information as you can in writing so you can refer back to it more than just once. Identify reliable websites and reading materials; several are included in this book. And keep asking questions until you feel confident that you have a good grasp of everything you need to understand your condition. Remember, there are no stupid questions, and no one can expect you to know all there is to know about herpes.

Fear

Are you afraid that no one will ever want you as a sexual partner now that you have herpes? You may fear that after you tell them about your herpes, potential partners will reject you in favor of someone who's uninfected. You fear the unknown: what will future outbreaks be like, how will you know when you're infectious, will you be able to identify herpes outbreaks when they happen, or will you infect family members through normal household living? Some people even fear that herpes will shorten their lives, but herpes doesn't affect life span, so you can take that particular concern off your list right away.

Others fear that they'll be "outed": that they'll tell someone who'll say something to others, and soon everyone will know. This is a reasonable concern but one over which you do have some degree of control; remember the previous chapter on telling others? If you're careful about whom you tell and ask those individuals to protect your privacy, you may manage to keep this matter to yourself and to those you want to know about it.

You may have irrational fears about infecting others through nonsexual means. Some of the most poignant letters I receive on the WebMD site are from parents who fear infecting their children through normal day-to-day activities of household living. For them, herpes is perceived as something awful that might befall their children through physical contact. But children don't get infected from parents who have genital herpes by typical household living experiences or by normal gestures of affection.

Finding out more about herpes lessens the fear. The unknown can be very scary, so instead of avoiding thinking or learning about herpes, dive right in. Immerse yourself in knowledge from accurate sources (see chapter 11). If you're staying home alone feeling stunned after finding out that you have herpes, use the time out to your advantage by educating yourself. You can also decrease your fear by trying out positive behaviors, like telling a potential partner that you have herpes. Yes, you might get rejected (that's certainly a possibility), but you'll at least know how it feels to tell someone. You'll discover that even if you're rejected, you'll survive the experience and the world won't come to an end, and perhaps you'll learn how to tell someone else a bit differently next time.

Embarrassment

Okay, I agree that your herpes diagnosis isn't something you'll want to post in your hometown paper. Having herpes can be "embarrassing." But what *is* embarrassment, really? In this case, it's probably concern about having attention called to private matters that you believe involve flaws in yourself. Embarrassment is related to shame but is felt on a much more superficial level.

Maybe you're embarrassed because the clinician you're seeing for this diagnosis delivered your child or has taken care of you since you started getting physical exams for Little League. You believe this particular problem just isn't one your clinician would expect to happen to you. But remember our discussion of how common genital herpes is? Your clinician sees it all the time, and your infection, though embarrassing to you, is routine for medical professionals. Instead of judging you as you might suspect, most sincerely care more about your emotional pain and how to minimize it. So don't give in to your discomfort and avoid discussing herpes with your health care provider. Push through, and ask for help to get you through this difficult time.

SUSTAINED EMOTIONAL REACTIONS

After you've had herpes for a few weeks or months, the emotions surrounding it sometimes change. You might still have some of the initial ones we talked about, but they'll tend to fade a bit as you get more information about herpes, in general, and your case, in particular. But now, some new feelings might come into play. Again, not everyone will experience all of what follows. You might move directly into accepting your condition, incorporate the reality of having herpes into your relationships, and get your life right back on track after negotiating this little jog in the road. Or you might be one who struggles a little more with it. Let's talk about some of the reactions to genital herpes that can come after the initial reactions have passed.

Loss

Having herpes can mean the loss of the part of your sexuality that was carefree and without restrictions. You now need to disclose that you have herpes to current and potential sex partners, and that's, at best, simply not much fun. But in these days of HIV and hepatitis, maybe it's not such a bad thing to get into the testing and telling mode with partners. In any case, this loss of feeling carefree about sexuality can be a struggle.

There's another kind of loss, that of your perception of yourself as unflawed. Maybe you haven't seen yourself as unflawed until you received your herpes diagnosis, but many people have, especially very young individuals who've not yet had enough life experience to know that no one is perfect. Getting herpes may be the first significant thing that's ever happened to you that's identified you as less than pristine. But the reality is that you were never flawless to begin with; no one is. It's easy enough to give lip service to that statement, but having something like herpes that's visible and not open to debate really brings home your "fallibility."

A third kind of loss, and it can be a big one, is the loss of control. Having herpes, you can't ever really know exactly when you're infectious to others, and that can be troubling. Your awareness of asymptomatic viral shedding takes away the control you may have thought you had to be able to avoid sex only when you have no symptoms in order to be "noninfectious." However, you now know that you can transmit herpes to your partner even when you're not having an outbreak. That awareness can cause the feeling of loss of control over your ability to have sex during certain "free times." You now know that you don't enjoy such a luxury.

Stigma

People who have genital herpes can feel socially stigmatized. Stigma relates to how society perceives others, and frankly, society sometimes doesn't treat genital herpes very kindly. There are the rude jokes about herpes that circulate. In the midst of a herpes joke, it's not easy to speak up and say, "I don't think herpes jokes are very funny; it's a common disease, and some people here could be infected, so let's joke about something else." Not everyone has negative feelings about people with herpes, but you still may be reluctant to disclose your infection status to others, because they may perceive you in a negative light simply due to your disease.

You can deal best with stigma by asking yourself, is the social negativity about genital herpes really warranted considering the minor medical severity of the disease, or is its "bad reputation" vastly overblown? I think you already know the answer, right? There's quite frankly little relationship between how herpes is perceived and the real medical problems it presents.

Shame

Shame is distress we feel about something we've done, but it's deeper than that; it's also about who we are. Feeling shame usually arises from standards we've been taught and the conflict we feel when our behavior is inconsistent with our beliefs and values. People who feel shame have feelings of disgrace, dishonor, and self-condemnation. The shame involved with herpes often comes from having engaged in a sexual encounter that we regret more than from having the disease itself. It's about our looking inside ourselves, as opposed to allowing ourselves to be judged by a society that's looking in on us. Shame contributes directly to problems with self-esteem. It can also contribute to problem behaviors like striking out at others or diverting blame to someone else to make us feel better, though that exercise rarely works. Some people attempt to deal with their shame by being overly pleasant or self-sacrificing to others to counteract their feelings of unworthiness, or they might try to achieve perfection in other areas of their lives to lessen the shame they feel about having herpes. But such compensatory behaviors can't get to the heart of the matter, so they rarely make shame disappear.

You'll feel less shame by learning to accept yourself, warts and all (no pun intended). Self-esteem is feeling positive about yourself, but self-acceptance is a broader and healthier condition. If you can learn to accept yourself with all of your limitations and flaws (herpes perhaps being a minor one in the big picture), decide that you're worthwhile regardless of the errors you make, and strive to be more consistent with your own expectations, shame can slide back into the shadows.

Isolation

People diagnosed with herpes sometimes pull inside themselves. Feeling shame can contribute to the desire to be alone and result in avoiding others, removing yourself from social situations, and feeling as if you're better off not having to face people with the truth about your disease or the dreaded "talk." Some people feel unworthy of interacting with others and mistakenly believe that they're no longer "good enough" to interact with others because of the infection. They may choose to avoid their friends or family, rather than have to share what's really bothering them.

In fact, it's perfectly okay to want to be by yourself for a little while. You need time to process what's happened and to feel a little shock, sadness, loss, and embarrassment. If you felt absolutely nothing, I'd be really concerned. Normal people don't get the news that they have a lifelong sexually transmitted infection, shrug their shoulders, and say, "Okay, what's next on the agenda?" We humans react, and for some people, that can require a little "quiet time." But when the "quiet time" stretches into weeks and months, when you refuse to see friends or family or to get involved with social activities, you should consider nudging yourself to get back into the world of the living, little by little.

Depression

Most people who get genital herpes don't suffer from clinical depression. You may feel shocked and upset, but almost everyone works his or her way back to normal psychological functioning within three to six months (Wald et al. 2005). However, you might get stuck in the sadness, shame, and loss aspects and not bounce back all that well. For most people, this isn't really a case of clinical depression either; it's just feeling down. For some, however, things can degrade into a truly depressed state of mind where life starts to look very bleak. How do you know if you're clinically depressed? An experienced clinician can best determine that, but there are some specific warning signs for depression. Please go over this checklist to see if many of these symptoms apply to you:

_____ Are you persistently sad?

_____ Do you feel pessimistic about the future?

_____ Do you feel like a failure?

_____ Do you feel guilty?

_____ Do you feel as if you're being punished?

_____ Do you dislike yourself?

_____ Are you critical of yourself?

_____ Do you cry a lot?

_____ Are you irritable?

_____ Have you lost interest in social activities?

_____ Are you having a hard time making decisions?

_____ Do you feel unattractive?

_____ Are you often tired for no physical reason?

_____ Have you lost interest in sex?

_____ Have you lost your appetite?

_____ Do you have trouble getting motivated to work?

_____ Have you lost interest in things that you previously enjoyed?

_____ Do you have trouble sleeping?

_____ Do you sometimes think you'd be better off dead?

If you checked off several of these questions, it's possible that you're clinically depressed. Many people recently diagnosed with herpes also answer yes to many of these questions, but these feelings don't usually persist over time. And there are degrees to the answers. All of us have felt tired, found it hard to work, or had trouble sleeping at some point, but if these issues start dominating what you do and how you feel every day, you need help. A qualified mental health professional can perform an assessment to find out if you're suffering from clinical depression. If you are, there are talk therapies, preferably cognitive behavioral therapy (which has been proven to work very well with this kind of problem), and medications to help you find your way out (Mindel 1996; McLarnon and Kaloupek 1988).

And no matter how badly you feel about having genital herpes, it's most certainly not a reason to kill yourself. If you have such thoughts in your head and any sort of plan to take your life, put this book down, pick up the phone, and seek professional help immediately. After all, we're talking about a minor infection that most people learn to manage and then lead fulfilled lives that include rich relationships. If you see death as the best answer, then this is one of those times in which you need help from a professional—now!

Relief

"Relief?" you ask. "Terri, what were you smoking when you wrote this book?" But some people do feel relief on hearing a herpes diagnosis, and a few of you are saying right now, "Aha, that's me!" Let's say you're in a relationship in which one person is infected and the other isn't. For years you've used condoms, examined genitals for signs and symptoms before having sex, stopped in the middle of sex if you felt any twinges, and were otherwise saintly in all your efforts to avoid transmitting herpes. And I suspect that one of you was a lot more worried about transmission than the other. But then "it" happened, and now you both have herpes. There's now a little place in your heart (and maybe even a big place in the hearts of some) that's relieved that you no longer have to do all that "stuff" to reduce the risk of transmission. This can be particularly true for couples who want to get pregnant at some point. They may be relieved about no longer facing the risk of transmitting herpes during the perilous third trimester.

Another kind of "relief" might be that you don't have something worse, like HIV infection or hepatitis C, that can actually shorten your life. Or you may have had troubling symptoms for years and gone to specialists to find out what was wrong with you. You've taken multiple medications, none of which worked, and had lab tests and diagnostic workups that yielded nothing. Now, finally, you have a clear diagnosis and a way to treat a relatively simple infection. You may not be jumping for joy, but you're relieved to know what's actually going on inside your body and to have effective medicines to treat a mostly benign medical problem.

Many people feel that herpes has had a positive influence on their lives. Some say that they make better decisions about their sex partners, others keep a closer watch on their general health habits, and others state that they're more careful to reduce the risk of acquiring HIV. I bet that if you think about it, you'll discover aspects of having genital herpes that are positive as well.

Decreased Self-Esteem

So often, I've had patients tell me they feel "one down" from people who don't have herpes. You may feel that if others had a choice about a partner, they'd always pick a person without herpes over you. You may have found adjectives to describe how you feel about yourself that include words like "dirty," "worthless," "slutty," "flawed," or "disgusting." I hesitated to even list these words, because I don't want you to get the idea that you should feel any of these things about yourself. Perhaps, however, you were already there. But put those words away right now. They don't describe you. This virus didn't conduct some kind of personality inventory to measure your worth or count the number of sexual partners you had in your life before it invaded your body. It just looked for a cell in which to live. Stop giving it so much power!

Now here are some tips for dealing with common negative thoughts that could be impacting your self-esteem.

RETHINKING YOUR FEELINGS

Where do feelings come from, anyway? There are many answers to that question, but since you're reading my book, I'll give you mine. Our emotional reactions, like the ones we just discussed, come not only from the events that take place in our lives but also from how we think about those events.

Let's say that two people get fired from their jobs. One person says, "I'm a total failure. I'll never find another job. After I use up my savings, I'll end up on the streets; I just know it. This is the end for me!" That person will feel desperation and despair. The other person thinks, "Well, that's a bummer. I liked that job, but it wasn't a perfect fit, I guess. I'll bet there are jobs out there that are better for me. I'll live on my savings, sell a few things, and take this opportunity to find something I like even better." The second person will feel a loss but will also feel hopeful that the future might be even better than the past.

The event is the same: being fired from a job. But the two individuals' thoughts about it couldn't be more different. And as a result, their feelings as they face unemployment are also very different. This is true about most of life's experiences. Take divorce. The event is the same for everyone—legal papers, new homes, living without a partner—but the thoughts and feelings vary widely from person to person. For the person who thinks daily about having the freedom to live as he or she wishes, the prospect of divorce might be welcome, but for the person who thinks that divorce is terrible and should be avoided at all costs, any feelings he or she has about the event will be extremely negative.

Right now, I'm going to try to help you think differently so that you can feel better. Since I've seen herpes patients for many years, I've noted some common thinking traps that many people with herpes fall into. This is not to say that you should be emotionally flat or cheerful about having herpes; that isn't realistic and doesn't make sense. But by thinking differently, perhaps you can turn around some negative feelings so that you can rediscover your happier self.

The three common thinking problems that I've identified are:

- Overgeneralizing
- Catastrophizing
- Demanding

And here are some of the destructive thoughts associated with these problem-thinking categories and some positive alternatives to try considering instead.

Overgeneralizing

Destructive thought: *"I'm worth less as a person, because I have genital herpes."* This type of thinking causes problems, because it involves identifying with your herpes: *"I am my herpes."*

Constructive alternative: *"My worth as a person is not affected by having herpes. I'm a person with many different characteristics, some positive and some negative. Herpes is only one characteristic, not all of me."*

At times, particularly during outbreaks, you may find it harder to accept yourself, and instead feel as if you're less desirable and less attractive. Having herpes may dominate your thoughts, making it harder for you to remember your better attributes. But they're there; just keep reminding yourself of them. List your strengths. No, you aren't perfect, but you weren't flawless before you had herpes either. People are drawn to you or move away from you for a variety of reasons; herpes is only one of many. Having herpes will challenge you to build on your strengths and motivate you to look honestly at your shortcomings too.

Destructive thought: *"I will* never *find anyone who'll want to be sexual with me, because I have herpes."* This belief generalizes from the present and attempts to predict the entire future with no evidence to support its conclusion. In short, you have no proof that you won't meet people who can accept the risk of getting herpes from you.

Constructive alternative: *"Why should I think that I'll never have healthy, long-term, sexual relationships? Some people may not want to take the risk of getting herpes, but there are most likely those who will, especially if the relationship is a good one."*

When some people are first diagnosed with herpes, they swear they'll never have sex again, that the risk of being rejected by someone is simply too great to bear. If you think this way, it suggests that there's no way you could stand it if you were rejected. But what about a life in which you remained completely alone? Wouldn't that, in the long run, be much more difficult than risking a possible rejection, if, of course, you desire to have a partner? How would it feel to be eighty-five and all alone, looking back and saying, "Well, at least I didn't give anyone small blisters on their genitals that flared up once in a while?" The reality is that once you begin including sex as part of your life, it's very hard to simply stop being sexual. The frustrations and emotional conflicts that arise as a result of trying to become celibate due to herpes are probably worse than having the infection. It's important to remember that the fears about transmitting herpes will ease with time, and a realistic plan to prevent transmission will replace the fears.

Destructive thought: *"Let's say I'm honest with a potential sexual partner, who turns out to be willing to be with me despite the small risk of herpes transmission. I'd still be a terrible person if I passed along herpes and ruined someone else's life forever. I could never forgive myself for this."* This negative belief is an example of *excessive* responsibility for another person's right to make choices. It also assumes that herpes would be *devastating* to your partner.

Constructive alternative: *"A full life involves risk taking. While I'd be deeply disappointed and sorry if an informed sexual partner contracted herpes from me, it would simply not be* all my fault. *In fact, it wouldn't be anyone's 'fault.' Other people have the right to make their own choices and take risks. Besides, herpes doesn't have to devastate others' lives. My partner has the right to choose to take the risk of getting herpes from me; this is a mutual decision, not mine alone."*

Transmitting herpes isn't the only risk that you'll take in the course of a relationship. You also risk losing someone to an incompatibility in personalities. There are risks that you'll grow apart over time, risks that issues like money, children, and sex will lead you into conflicts you just can't solve. The list is long, and herpes is only one item on that list.

Catastrophizing

Destructive thought: *"Having herpes is the end of my world. I'll never, ever be happy again."* This belief usually implies that having herpes is simply too much to bear and that one cannot possible be happy in spite of having herpes.

Constructive alternative: *"Having herpes is certainly inconvenient and an unfortunate hassle. But other people manage to find happiness in spite of having herpes, and so can I."*

If you really think that having herpes is a catastrophe, keep getting more information about the disease. The more you know, the better you'll be able to cope. Seeing a mental health counselor may also be helpful. Having a close friend to talk to is also very useful, because keeping all of your thoughts inside can make you feel pretty lonely.

Demanding

Destructive thought: *"I* should not *have contracted herpes, and my partner* should not *have given it to me."* These thoughts jump from the realistic regret about not having avoided getting herpes to the unrealistic demand that such an undesirable thing *must* not have happened. Remember that most people who have genital herpes don't know it. People can't prevent the transmission of something they don't know they have. And let's imagine that you got herpes from a casual sexual encounter. Where is your responsibility in this? Did you even ask your partner to get tested for STIs prior to having sex, and were you also tested?

Constructive alternative: *"I wish I'd not contracted herpes, but at the time I got it, I was unaware that my partner could give it to me. I did the best I could, given the information I had at the time, and perhaps I should've had more. In similar future circumstances, I'll do better."*

This thought allows you to share in the responsibility and gives you credit for doing the best that you could while encouraging you to do better next time. Accepting responsibility for any part you played in getting herpes can help you leave behind destructive demanding thoughts.

Destructive thought: *"I* should *not have to deal with the pain, discomfort, and practical problems associated with herpes."* This thought also insists that one's preference for not having to endure misfortune *must* be granted. But why must it be granted? Where is it written that you shouldn't have any pain or problems in life? Are you somehow different from all other people on this planet who do have problems to some degree?

Constructive alternative: *"I certainly don't like dealing with the disadvantages of having herpes, but life sometimes deals us 'unfair' blows. It's just part of the human experience to have to go through things that we don't like very much. And there are plenty of people out there with medical problems that are far more serious than mine.*

"This isn't going to be the last bad thing that happens in my life, and if I can learn to take this one in stride, it'll be good practice for things to come that are far more serious."

You certainly don't have to use the specific constructive alternatives suggested above to replace the self-defeating ones, but it's important that you come up with your own believable, helpful ways of thinking about the problems around having herpes. To accept the helpful beliefs and drop the unhelpful ones, I recommend the following three actions:

- Try to see that the helpful thoughts are actually more reasonable and rational than the unhelpful ones.

- Remind yourself frequently that the unhelpful thoughts lead to emotional distress, while the helpful ones create emotions that help you achieve your goal. You may have to focus on the constructive thought several times a day, but if you do so long enough, it'll become a sincerely held belief, not one that you have to work at accepting.

- Act in accordance with the more helpful beliefs. This involves facing the discomfort of risking beginning new relationships, if you're currently unattached. It involves *not* becoming reclusive or acting as if you don't deserve the benefits of sex and intimacy.

PSYCHOSEXUAL PROBLEMS

Sometimes people with genital herpes develop new problems with sexual performance. Men may have difficulty achieving and keeping erections or may ejaculate too quickly during intercourse. Women may have difficulty becoming aroused and lubricated or in achieving orgasm. Often, these issues are a direct result of worrying about herpes transmission while being sexual with a partner. You might not be aware of the worried thoughts that lead to such problems, but often they're there. Men might subconsciously think that if they don't have an erection, intercourse isn't possible, so they therefore can't infect their partners with herpes. An uninfected partner might be turned off by the subliminal concern about potentially getting infected, which turns off the sexual response. Premature ejaculation also works along these lines. If the penis is inside a partner for only a short period of time and one ejaculates quickly, the risk of transmission is lower and the virus is less likely to spread (or so the subconscious, fearful thinking goes). If someone is worrying a great deal about transmitting a disease, it's hard to focus on the feelings, both physical and emotional, surrounding lovemaking to achieve an orgasm.

The key to resolving these problems probably lies in talking openly and gently about them with your partner. Good communication skills are an invaluable aid.

In summary, herpes itself may involve physical discomfort and impose certain restrictions on your spontaneity. Many people experience a variety of intense emotions when they first find out they have herpes, but shock, anger, sadness, fear, and confusion are normal feelings. Later on, you may feel stigmatized, isolated, depressed, anxious, and unworthy. If you become significantly depressed or immobilized with fear of the future, there are effective ways of combating these difficult emotions and regaining your confidence by seeking professional help. Identify the beliefs that are hurting you, and make a concerted effort to change them. Sometimes problems with sexual performance can come up related to herpes transmission. All of these problems are solvable with time, perspective, and new ways of thinking about having genital herpes.

QUESTIONS AND ANSWERS ON THE PSYCHOLOGICAL IMPACT OF HERPES

I just found out last week that I have genital herpes. The pain of the lesions and the pain of peeing are incredible, and I can't do anything but cry. I've taken the whole week off from work, so I've lost half of my vacation time for the year—all because some jerk didn't tell me he had herpes. I feel as if I'm drowning in pain, anger, and sadness. Of course you do. All of those feelings are completely normal, and if you felt anything less, I'd be surprised. One thing you might want to do right away is get the pain under control. Ask your clinician for prescription pain medicine. If there's ever a good time for using heavy-duty pain medication, this is it. Also, look back in chapter 6 for tips for dealing with symptoms like pain while urinating. Pain greatly influences how you see your situation, and once you get some relief, either through medicine or as the lesions heal naturally, you'll start to feel better. But even then, this is a huge change for you, and it doesn't sound as if the person who gave you herpes is someone you'd turn to for support. I hope you have others around you whom you can tell and who can help you feel loved and cared for. Give yourself lots of time. It'll get better for you, but give it months, not days. Talk to others who have the same problem, if you can; let them support you, and let your clinician know what you're going through emotionally, if you feel you'd find an "open" ear. This is all so fresh and raw; just try to make it through this dark period, and things will start looking brighter later.

I'm a woman who's had HSV 1 genitally for five years and was with the woman who gave it to me until a couple of months ago, when she broke up with me. After I was diagnosed, it didn't seem like such a big deal: she was infected, and so was I; and I've had only a couple of outbreaks, so that wasn't an issue either. But now I have to tell people, and I'm freaking out! What seemed like nothing before is now huge. What can I do? Your HSV 1 genital infection is still the same, so there's nothing different there. It's how you have to think about it that's different now, right?—and whom you have to tell. There are probably several things going on here at once; you were with someone for a long time who recently left you, and that's probably an emotional load to carry. When you were with her and she also had HSV 1, it felt okay, because there was no risk, no need to tell, and few outbreaks. I'd bet you didn't even think much about herpes when you were with her. But now, that safe environment is gone, so in many ways, you're probably feeling pretty exposed. Remember that genital HSV 1 is infrequently shed from your body and is less likely to be infectious to others. Also, if you meet someone new who already has cold sores or an HSV 1 positive antibody test, your infection really doesn't need to be an issue at all. Take your time in getting to know someone before you share this. You're very newly out of a long-term relationship, so you may want to go slowly about getting into a new sexual relationship anyway.

I've only had two partners in my life. I'm thirty years old, and it was my second partner who gave me genital herpes. I've been so careful about sex! My religious background is very strict and conservative, and I never should've had sex until I got married anyway. I get that now, but it's too late. I'd give anything to go back and do this over again. No one will want me now that I'm ruined with this virus. I'm never going to date again or put myself in a position to be rejected because of this awful disease. Do you suppose that there might be others in your religion who've also had sex outside of marriage and who've lived in a way that isn't completely consistent with all of the teachings you grew up with? I'd say with certainty that there are! People are fallible; they slide out of "perfect" ways and make errors, but most go on. And so will you. I know you have herpes, but what are some of the other qualities that you have? If I asked you to write down five things that you consider to be your strengths, what would you write? Are any of them characteristics that others would find attractive? And what if the shoe were on the other foot? What if you met someone who'd made an error and who was living with a similar problem? How would you view that? Would you reject that person because of it? Or would you consider that problem in light of the total person he or she is? I believe that's what people will do with you, if you'll give them that chance. And herpes isn't an awful disease. You perceive it as awful right now, given all the circumstances, but it's really just annoying—uncomfortable but manageable. So while you're listing your strengths, try also to change the negative terms you've been using to think about herpes.

My girlfriend has genital herpes. She told me about it before we had sex, and I got it from her about a month ago. So far, I'm doing okay with it. I love her, she loves me, sex is still great with us, and herpes just doesn't seem to be that big of a deal. I read all this stuff about depression, suicidal thoughts, and shame, and I'm wondering if I'm missing something here. Should I be more upset about this? No, you aren't missing anything. I talk about all those negative emotions because many people experience them, but not everyone does. You're in a loving relationship, you knew you were taking a risk, and you've accepted what's happened and what you can't change. That's great. However, if your situation with your partner ever changes, you might see the situation differently then, but maybe not. I'm glad you're doing so well.

I had a six-month affair (I've been married for twenty years) and got HSV 2 from my lover. My wife and I still have sex, I haven't told her about the herpes, and obviously I can't just start using condoms out of the clear blue sky, because she'd wonder what was going on. I know it's going to kill her to get this news, and I don't want to hurt her. What am I going to do? I think you can start by being honest with yourself. Sure, she'll be hurt, but one of the reasons you don't want to tell her is because of how her reaction will impact you. She will probably be very angry and devastated, might not want to have sex with you, and could maybe even leave you. And you wouldn't like any of that; no one would. But I can guarantee that if she gets herpes from you because you didn't tell her that you're infected, she'll be even more upset. Let's see, would it be better for her to get herpes from you before you tell or to allow her to make some informed decisions? Put yourself in her position. What would you want? My advice is to stop having sex with her right now, muster up the courage to tell her about the affair and the herpes, and ask for her forgiveness for the significant error you've made. Have her tested for HSV, and if she's uninfected and still wants to continue your sexual relationship, get on daily therapy and use condoms, at least for now. But be prepared for a sexual "vacation," at best. Affairs are one thing, but getting herpes from an affair is essentially like having that affair tag along with your marriage for the rest of your lives. It's very tough, and I think you can expect some challenging days ahead in your marriage.

My girlfriend has herpes, and I don't (we did the blood antibody tests). She's on daily medication, and I use condoms when we have sex. We've been together for nine months. I've tried and tried to move past thinking about her herpes, and instead of getting less worried over time, I'm getting more worried. If she had cancer, I could handle that like a champ, but this—this is so different; I just don't want to get it! I think about it every time we have sex, and often, I have trouble getting an erection from worrying about the herpes, so the condom thing doesn't work very well. Then she starts crying and feeling unattractive, and I can't tell her what I'm really worried about, because then she'll feel bad about her herpes. I know I should feel lucky to have such a nice girlfriend; she's so good to me and we get along, but as hard as I've tried, I can't get past this. I feel like a real bum about this, but it is what it is. What can I do? I'm going to suggest a couples counselor for the two of you so you can examine your specific fears about getting herpes and learn to communicate more openly with your partner about what's going on inside your head. Counseling may not help you. Some people just can't put this aside and move on with a relationship. It doesn't make you a bad person (just as her having herpes doesn't make her a bad person) if you can't move past this. It just means that this is an area where logic might not overcome your fears about herpes. But please try talking with a professional. Even if counseling can't help you work out your relationship, it may help your partner come out of this stronger and less hurt. And it may help you see some vulnerable areas in yourself that could use some work. And here's a thought for the future: get testing for STIs with partners before you have sex, and if they have herpes, consider moving on right away.

I contracted herpes about a month ago from a guy I'm no longer with. I'm completely immobilized by this news. Yes, I work, but I avoid friends and just hang out with my dog. I feel that if people could really see what's inside of me, they'd go, "Ick! I don't want to be around her with that *disease."* I think a herpes support group is just the thing for you. There, or online, you can meet other people who are going through what you're going through. You can talk to other people with herpes without feeling as if they'll say, "Ick!" because everyone is in the same boat. You can go to one of the online dating services or chat areas listed in chapter 11 and just talk to people. You don't need to date; just talk. Share the feelings that you're having. I think you desperately need to open up to someone and share what you're going through. Besides, when you talk with someone who's had herpes for a while, you'll learn that time does heal and that there's life after herpes for you too.

Chapter 9

HIV and HSV 2: Things Could Be More Complicated

In the United States, 60 to 70 percent of HIV-positive people are also infected with HSV 2 (Schacker 2001). These two viruses are closely intertwined but not in a good way for the person who has both infections. But which is the chicken and which is the egg?

There's a good chance that herpes came first. A person who has HSV 2 genital infection is two to five times more likely to acquire HIV infection (but this doesn't apply to genital HSV 1, which has a very different recurrence and shedding pattern) (Freeman et al. 2006). And if you have new HSV 2 infection, as opposed to an established infection, the risk is even higher, because as we know, HSV 2 is more active when it's new (Abu-Raddad et al. 2008). "Well," you say, "it's easy enough to understand why; the same behaviors that put people at risk for herpes put them at risk for HIV." But you'd be only partially correct. If you compare the HIV acquisition risks for individuals who are the same age, have the same number of sexual partners, and use or don't use condoms with similar frequency, those who have HSV 2 are far more likely to get HIV. In other words, HSV 2 is an independent risk factor for getting HIV infection. So why is that?

BROKEN SKIN

When you have HSV 2 genital infection, you give off virus from your body in a process known as shedding. By definition, that means virus is leaving your body, which it does either during obvious outbreaks (through breaks in the skin that are big enough to see) or by microscopic asymptomatic shedding through little tiny breaks in the skin. Most herpes virus shedding is without symptoms. Yet the skin breaks, whether large or small, allow HIV to get into the body more easily if it's around. Let's clarify something right away: HIV doesn't float down through the air and seep into your underwear to infect you. You have to be having sex with someone who's HIV infected for it to be a risk to you. If you're having sex only with someone who's HIV negative (and you both should know that through testing, not by assuming or guessing), then you can stop reading right here until you or your partner adds or changes partners.

CD4 T CELLS TO THE RESCUE

Another reason why herpes puts you at increased risk of HIV infection is the kind of immune response your body uses to deal with active herpes virus, either through an outbreak or asymptomatic shedding. When your herpes is active on the genital skin or mucosa, your body alerts a specific immune cell called a *CD4 T cell*. That kind of cell receives the message: "Go to the genitals quickly; that pesky herpes virus is back!" So the CD4 T cells migrate to the site of viral reactivation to defend against the herpes outbreak or shedding. Unfortunately, it just so happens that CD4 T cells are the very ones that HIV prefers to infect. So it could be the perfect storm: there's a break in your skin, either microscopic or obvious, that leaves it open to attack. HIV-vulnerable CD4 T cells get recruited to the area by the immune system to aid in resolving the active herpes virus at the site of broken skin. If HIV is present and you add in the friction of sexual activity to the whole picture, you can see why T cells can be far more easily infected with HIV when you have HSV 2.

The Police Car Analogy

Having trouble picturing all of this in your head? Imagine it this way: Think of the CD4 T cell as a powerful police car, gliding through the bloodstream, waiting for messages from central command about where it's needed next. Imagine the herpes virus as a vandal whose claim to fame is making holes in walls and doing other minor damage. Imagine the genital skin as the wall that's vulnerable to the damage of the vandals, and imagine the herpes reactivation (whether an obvious outbreak or an asymptomatic shedding episode with a break in the skin) as the hole that's been made by the vandal. When the herpes virus becomes active, central command tells the CD4 T cell police car that there's been another attack on the wall; it needs to go to the breech to deal with the vandals. Only, waiting outside the wall are the *really* bad guys, HIV terrorists. And they *love* to hijack police cars—their favorite cars to steal. And what they really like to do while riding in the stolen police car is jump in the back seat and make more of themselves! So the CD4 T cell (the police car) speeds to the hole in the wall (herpes reactivation) to arrest the vandal (the HSV 2 virus). The real bad guys (the HIV intruders) see the police car pull up to the hole in the wall, jump in, take over the car, and begin rapidly reproducing as the police car (CD4 T cell) speeds back into town, effectively setting up HIV infection in the whole body. Had the vandals not banged a hole in the wall, the CD4 T police car wouldn't have gotten the message to respond, and the HIV terrorists wouldn't have entered the body so easily.

TREATING HSV 2 TO PREVENT HIV?

So, if you want the wall to stay intact, you go on daily suppressive antiviral therapy, right? That's what researchers from the University of Washington thought. Large studies were done in Africa, Peru, and the United States, placing women and gay men who were HSV 2 positive and HIV negative on either 400 milligrams of acyclovir twice a day or a placebo to see if the medication reduced the risk of HIV infection. However, no benefit was seen for the drug over the placebo (Celum et al. 2008). The results were certainly disappointing and also surprising. Why did herpes medicine fail to reduce the risk of HIV infection? There's no clear answer. The subjects took the medicine as directed, and fewer genital sores were seen in the acyclovir-treated subjects, but HIV acquisition rates were the same. One takeaway message is, if you have genital HSV 2, you should have your sex partners tested for HIV. If they're positive, be very careful with your sexual activity.

WHAT IF YOU'RE HIV AND HSV 2 POSITIVE?

What if you're HIV positive and you also have genital HSV 2? Your herpes may be more difficult to control, especially if your CD4 T count is low (less than 350). Your herpes outbreaks could last longer and be more severe. You'll benefit from taking suppressive therapy to reduce viral shedding and better control outbreaks. In addition, daily therapy will help reduce your risk of transmitting HIV to others, since HIV can be carried with the herpes virus to sexual partners. Taking daily therapy for herpes will reduce the amount of HIV in your bloodstream and, for women, in genital secretions (Nagot et al. 2008). It's important to consult your HIV health care provider to ensure that your herpes is as well managed as your HIV infection.

Chapter 10

Other STIs: There Are *More*!

You might be wondering why I use the term "STI" or "sexually transmitted infection" rather than "sexually transmitted disease" ("STD"). The terminology has changed in recent years to fit our understanding of what's going on with sexually communicable illnesses. The word "disease" implies that symptoms are present, while an "infection" can be present without any symptoms at all, and herpes is the perfect example most of the time: the virus is in your body, and even if you never notice any manifestations, the infection can still be passed to other people. It's a medical distinction that may not seem important to you, and if you'd like to still use "STD," that's fine, because I often slip into that as well. But the most current terminology for viruses, bacteria, and so on that are passed from one person to another through sexual contact is "infection" rather than "disease."

Herpes isn't the only STI out there, of course, and it's definitely *not* the most dangerous, just the most maligned. Certain STIs can cause infertility, cancers, and even death. There are many good reasons to practice safer sex, and I'm about to tell you about twelve of those. Bacteria, viruses, fungi, protozoa, and skin bugs can all cause STIs. There are about twenty-eight that are officially considered STIs, but these are the twelve most commonly found in the United States. An excellent resource for information on STIs is the Centers for Disease Control and Prevention website: www.cdc.gov/STD.

VIRAL INFECTIONS

The STIs caused by viruses are the fastest growing group, probably because we're gaining ground on bacterial infections with effective antibiotics, but we have fewer tools to treat or cure viral infections. We've already covered herpes, which would go under this heading, so let's move on to wart virus, more formally known as HPV.

Human Papillomavirus (HPV): What Is It?

Genital human papillomavirus (HPV) is the most frequently acquired STI in the nation. Over forty HPV types infect the skin and mucous membranes of the genital tract in men and women, including the skin of the penis, vulva, anus, cervix, and rectum. Most people who become infected with HPV don't even know they have it. Genital HPV is passed on to others through genital contact, which includes vaginal and anal intercourse, and genital-to-genital rubbing, even if actual penetration doesn't occur. A person can have HPV infection even if years have passed since he or she had sex. Most people who have HPV don't know they're infected or that they're passing the virus to sex partners.

HPV types are often referred to as "low risk" (external wart causing) or "high risk" (cancer causing). Specific types of HPV cause external genital warts in men and women. Other HPV types can cause cervical cancer and other cancers of the vulva, vagina, anus, penis, mouth, and throat. The types of HPV that cause external genital warts are *not* the same as the types that cause cervical cancer. If you have genital warts, don't jump to the conclusion that you're going to get cancer.

Fifty to eighty percent of sexually active men and women acquire genital HPV infection at some point in their lives. But the good news is that 90 percent of HPV infections clear on their own within two years (Plummer et al. 2007).

Genital warts usually appear as small growths or groups of growths in the genital area. They can be raised or flat, singular or multiple, small or large, and sometimes the top of the growth has a cauliflower-like appearance. They can appear on the vulva; in or around the vagina or anus; or on the cervix, penis, scrotum, groin, or thigh. Warts usually appear within weeks or months after sexual contact with an infected person. If they don't get treated, genital warts might go away, stay and remain unchanged, or increase in size or number. They won't turn into cancer.

Cervical cancer is a sexually transmitted infection caused by HPV. It doesn't show symptoms until it's quite advanced, so it's very important for sexually active women to get screened regularly for cervical cancer with a Pap smear. Certain populations may be at higher risk for HPV-related cancers, such as gay and bisexual men, and individuals with weak immune systems (including those who have HIV or AIDS).

You can lower your chances of getting HPV by starting sexual activity later in life (it might be too late for that) and staying in a mutually monogamous relationship. Using condoms and avoiding smoking also reduce the risk of HPV infection. However, even people with only one lifetime sex partner can get HPV if their partners were infected with HPV from someone else before the sexual relationship began.

HPV Diagnosis

Genital warts are diagnosed by physical exam. The clinician looks for the characteristic growths in the genital area. It isn't always easy to distinguish warts from normal tissue, because some people just have bumps on their genitals. An experienced clinician can usually tell what's a wart and what isn't.

Cervical cell changes (early signs of cervical cancer) can be identified by a Pap smear. A second test that looks specifically for HPV can identify high-risk or low-risk HPV types on a woman's cervix, but this test is usually performed only on women over thirty, since younger women tend to clear HPV on their own.

Unfortunately, there's currently no approved test to find HPV in men.

HPV Treatment

Visible genital warts are treated by patient-applied medications such as Aldara (imiquimod) or condylox (podophilox) or by clinician-performed treatments (liquid nitrogen, trichloroacetic acid, or laser treatment). Most of those treatments destroy the warts' excess tissue. The topical treatment, Aldara, stimulates the body's immune response to fight the wart virus more effectively. Some people choose to forego treatment to see if the warts will disappear on their own. Many people require more than one office visit to treat their warts.

Cervical cancer is most treatable when diagnosed early. There are new forms of surgery, radiation therapy, and chemotherapy available. See www.cancer.org for more information. Women who get routine Pap testing can identify problems *before* cancer develops, and prevention is always better than treatment. Most cervical cancer is found in women who have never had a Pap smear or who haven't had one in the past five years.

HPV Vaccine

Gardasil, a vaccine, can now protect uninfected females from the four types of HPV that cause 70 percent of cervical cancers (types 16 and 18), and most external genital warts (types 6 and 11) and certain vaginal and vulvar cancers (FUTURE II Study Group 2007). The vaccine is FDA approved for females aged nine to twenty-six. This vaccine is safe and effective, and can eliminate 70 percent of the cervical-cancer risk in women who are not already infected with HPV (FUTURE II Study Group 2007). Even if a woman has had one type of HPV, the vaccine is still recommended to prevent the other types that she hasn't yet had. Very few women have had all four HPV types that the vaccine prevents. HPV vaccines not only reduce the risk of getting HPV infection, but they also reduce the number of expensive and invasive *LEEP* (loop electrical excision procedure; a procedure to remove dangerous cells from the cervix) and *colposcopy* (a method of looking for cervical abnormalities with a special microscope) procedures performed to investigate abnormal Pap smears. These procedures can be both expensive and invasive.

Side effects of the vaccine are mostly infection-site reactions, including redness, swelling, pain, and itching. The number of side effects from Gardasil is about half the average number reported for other vaccines.

A second vaccine, Cervarix, offers protection against two cervical cancer strains of the virus (type 16 and 18) but not the external wart virus strains (Paavonen et al. 2007). Cervarix is not yet FDA approved for use in the United States. At this writing, there's no vaccine licensed to prevent HPV-related diseases in men, but studies are under way.

Special note: HPV can infect areas that aren't covered by a condom, but condoms are still very effective, if not fully protective. The only sure way to prevent HPV completely is to avoid all sexual activity.

Hepatitis C: What Is It?

Hepatitis C virus (*HCV*) causes a serious, contagious liver disease. Approximately three million people in the United States have chronic HCV infection; it's most prevalent in people born between 1945 and 1965. The majority was infected during the 1970s and 1980s, when hepatitis C infection rates were highest (CDC 1998).

The illness can range in severity from a mild episode lasting for a few weeks to a serious, lifelong, or fatal condition. Hepatitis C is usually spread when blood from a person infected with the hepatitis C virus enters the body of someone who isn't infected. Sharing needles or other equipment to inject drugs is most often the way hepatitis C is transmitted, but it can also be spread sexually. The risk of transmission from sexual contact is low but increases for those who have multiple sex partners, have another STI, engage in rough sex, or are also infected with HIV.

For most people, the acute first infection leads to chronic, lifelong infection. However, of those who get hepatitis C, 20 to 40 percent clear the virus from their bodies without treatment and won't develop chronic infection (Soriano et al. 2008). Experts don't fully understand why this happens. The most severe chronic hepatitis C cases can result in liver cancers or death.

There's no vaccine for hepatitis C. The best way to prevent it is by avoiding behaviors that can spread the disease, especially injection-drug use.

Hepatitis C Diagnosis

Most people with chronic hepatitis C don't have symptoms and don't know that they're infected. However, if a person has been infected for many years, his or her liver may be damaged, and the infection is often discovered after abnormal liver function values from routine blood work are found during a physical exam.

Hepatitis C Treatment

People with hepatitis C are usually most effectively treated by an infectious-disease doctor or one who specializes in gastroenterology. Chronic hepatitis C patients should be monitored regularly for signs of liver disease and evaluated for treatment. The usual treatment is a combination of two medicines: interferon and ribavirin. However, not every person with chronic hepatitis C needs or will benefit from that treatment.

Hepatitis B: What Is It?

Hepatitis B can also cause liver disease, and is a different virus from hepatitis C. This virus is much more often sexually transmitted, but it can also be transferred through blood or body fluids, IV drug injection, and sometimes from mother to baby. It's very common in certain parts of the world but not as common in the United States, possibly because hepatitis B vaccination is part of the normal U.S. childhood immunization program, although that's only been the case since about 1981.

Hepatitis B Diagnosis

There are various blood antibody tests to diagnose hepatitis B, but I won't go into detail here, because it can be pretty complicated. Infected people might also get a noticeable first infection with hepatitis B: mild fevers; dark urine; vomiting; and yellow, itchy skin. Sometimes this first infection is severe, but it usually clears by itself without complications. If a person doesn't clear the infection and it becomes chronic, it can lead to severe liver problems like liver cancer.

Hepatitis B Treatment

Most often, people who get this infection don't need treatment; they resolve the symptoms on their own within several weeks. Occasionally, treatment is needed to stop the virus from replicating and to prevent further liver damage. A much better approach to hepatitis B is vaccination! The vaccine comes in a series of three injections and can be given in combination with the hepatitis A vaccine. All sexually active adults would potentially benefit from hepatitis B vaccination.

Molluscum Contagiosum: What Is It?

Molluscum contagiosum is a harmless, superficial skin condition caused by the poxvirus. The virus causes small white, pink, or flesh-colored bumps or growths that have a dimple or pit in the center. The bumps are usually smooth and firm, and, in most people, range in size from a pinhead to as large as a pencil eraser (two to five millimeters in diameter). They may appear anywhere on the body but most often, when sexually transmitted, are found in the pubic-hair area, on the shaft of the penis, or on the thighs. They usually disappear on their own within six to twelve months without treatment and without leaving scars, but during that time, they can multiply into hundreds of bumps if left untreated.

Molluscum is also sometimes found on children who attend day care centers, and it's not sexually transmitted in that situation. The virus is spread through skin-to-skin contact, from touching affected skin, or by touching a surface with the virus on it, such as a towel, clothing, or toys.

Molluscum Contagiosum Diagnosis

Molluscum is diagnosed most often by a clinician who's looking for the typical presentation: a flesh-colored bump with a dimple (*umbilication*) in the middle. The clinician can also nick the bump with a sterile needle and squeeze out the contents, which is like a thick cheese. Sometimes, a sample is sent to the lab for confirmation, but this is usually unnecessary.

Molluscum Contagiosum Treatment

Treatment for molluscum is usually recommended if the growths are in the genital area (on or near the penis, vulva, vagina, or anus), because they can multiply rapidly and be spread to others, and because most people just don't like the way they look.

Freezing the bumps with liquid nitrogen is one treatment option. Another is to remove the cheesy substance inside by squeezing the bumps, then cleaning the area with alcohol. It helps to nick the surface first to allow an escape route for the substance inside. Some clinicians also use Aldara to treat molluscum, and it works as well as it does for HPV. It's a good idea to stick with proven treatments rather than explore the Internet for answers to this minor but annoying skin problem.

Assuming there's no further contact with another infected person, once all the molluscum contagiosum bumps go away, new bumps shouldn't appear. Recovery from one infection with molluscum doesn't prevent future infections, however.

BACTERIAL INFECTIONS

Antibiotics treat the bacterial infections we'll discuss next. They're easily curable, but if left untreated, there can be serious consequences.

Syphilis: What Is It?

Syphilis is often called "the great imitator," because so many of its symptoms are similar to those of other diseases. Syphilis is passed through direct sexual contact with an infected person. Pregnant women can pass syphilis to their babies, but almost every pregnant woman is routinely tested for syphilis these days, so this isn't a major concern. Syphilis isn't spread through contact with inanimate objects like toilet seats.

The first stage of syphilis is usually the appearance of a single sore (called a *chancre*), but there can be multiple sores. The chancre is usually round and painless, with a raised edge that's firm to the touch. It lasts three to six weeks and heals without treatment. But if the infected person isn't treated, the infection progresses to the secondary stage.

The second-stage symptoms include a skin rash, sores, or both. The rash usually doesn't itch, and rashes can appear as the chancre sore is healing or several weeks later. The classic secondary syphilis rash is rough, red or reddish-brown spots that appear on the palms of the hands and soles of the feet. Sometimes it can show up in other places, like the chest or back. Other symptoms of secondary syphilis may include fever, swollen lymph glands, sore throat, patchy hair loss, headaches, weight loss, muscle aches, and fatigue. The symptoms go away with or without treatment, but without it, syphilis will still be in the body, and the infection will progress to the latent, and possibly late, stages of the disease.

The latent stage of syphilis begins when the primary and secondary symptoms end. Without treatment, the infected person continues to have syphilis even though there are no symptoms, and it can last for years. The late stages of syphilis develop in about 15 percent of people who've not been treated, and can appear ten to twenty years after first infection (CDC 2006). Late syphilis can damage internal organs, including the brain, nerves, eyes, heart, blood vessels, liver, bones, and joints. People with late-stage syphilis may have difficulty coordinating their muscle movements and experience paralysis, numbness, gradual blindness, dementia, and possibly death.

Syphilis Diagnosis

Syphilis is diagnosed in one of two ways: by examining material from a chancre using a dark-field microscope that can detect the actual *spirochete* (the bacteria) or by blood testing. There are two different blood tests done to confirm syphilis. One is a nonspecific test (RPR or VDRL) that can sometimes mistakenly pick up antibodies unrelated to syphilis (false positives). The second follow-up antibody test (FTA-ABS or MHA-TP) is much more specific for syphilis. Low levels of the specific antibodies usually stay in the blood for years, even after the disease has been successfully treated. If that happens, future blood tests will look for rises in the amount of antibody as an indication of true infection. Because untreated syphilis in a pregnant woman can infect and possibly kill her developing baby, every pregnant woman routinely has a blood test for syphilis.

Syphilis Treatment

Syphilis is most often treated and cured with injectable penicillin, unless the infected person is allergic to it, in which case other antibiotics can be substituted. The dose and frequency required depend upon how long the person has been infected.

Gonorrhea: What Is It?

I'll bet you've heard some of the slang names for *gonorrhea*: "the whites," "the drip," "a race horse" (because it's always running), "GC," and "the clap." Gonorrhea is another bacterial infection.

In women, it thrives in the warm, moist areas of the reproductive tract, including the cervix, fallopian tubes, anus, and urethra. It rarely infects the throat and eyes. Most infected women have no symptoms, and if symptoms are present, they're often mistaken for a bladder or vaginal infection. Symptoms might include pain or burning with urination, increased vaginal discharge, or vaginal bleeding between periods or after intercourse.

In men, gonorrhea can infect the penis, throat, eyes, and anus. Almost all men who have gonorrhea in their penises develop symptoms of the infection within two to five days after infection. Symptoms include a burning sensation when urinating and a large amount of white, yellow, or green discharge from the urethra. Some men get painful or swollen testicles, which indicates that the infection has become more serious. When men come to my clinic and tell me that they had to put toilet paper in their shorts to deal with the discharge on the trip to the office, almost without testing I know that they have gonorrhea.

For both men and women, symptoms of rectal infection may include discharge, anal itching, soreness, bleeding, painful bowel movements, or no symptoms at all. Gonorrhea infection in the throat may cause a sore throat but usually doesn't cause any other symptoms.

Gonorrhea Diagnosis

Gonorrhea is easily diagnosed by looking at a sample of the discharge under the microscope using a test called a *Gram's stain*. In the sample, the lab technician can see pus cells, and inside the pus cells, he or she can detect the gonorrhea bacteria that the pus cells have eaten. Not all clinics have the ability to do this rapid test, but testing can be done from a urine or swab sample that's sent to a lab.

Gonorrhea Treatment

Gonorrhea is currently most often treated with a single dose of the oral antibiotic, cefixime, though there are other oral antibiotics that also work well. The disease can be treated with injectable medicines, but that isn't usually necessary unless the infection has become more complicated. Because about half the people infected with gonorrhea simultaneously have chlamydia, antibiotics for both infections are given together (see the treatment for chlamydia in the next section). Some strains of gonorrhea are now resistant to certain antibiotics, so you should try to get confirmation that the treatment you'll receive for gonorrhea is the most up to date.

If gonorrhea is left untreated for a while, it can cause more serious problems, particularly in women. If gonorrhea moves into the upper genital tract (uterus and fallopian tubes), it can cause a syndrome called *pelvic inflammatory disease* (*PID*). PID can cause scarring of the fallopian tubes and make infertility more likely. Men can develop complications in the testicular area. If you have pelvic or testicular pain, please see a clinician right away.

Chlamydia: What Is It?

Chlamydia is a very common bacterial infection, especially in people in their teens and twenties (CDC 2006). Even though symptoms of chlamydia are usually mild or absent, serious complications can occur, including infertility, pelvic inflammatory disease, and tubal pregnancy. For this reason, federal guidelines suggest that all sexually active women under age twenty-six be screened annually for chlamydia (U.S. Preventive Services Task Force 2001).

Chlamydia is known as a "silent" disease, because about 75 percent of infected women and more than half of infected men report no symptoms at all (CDC 2007a).

In women, bacteria initially infect the cervix and the urethra. There might be an abnormal vaginal discharge or a burning sensation when urinating. When the infection spreads from the cervix to the fallopian tubes, some women develop lower abdominal pain, low back pain, nausea, fever, pain or bleeding during intercourse, or bleeding between menstrual periods.

Men may have a clear or cloudy discharge from the penis or a burning sensation when urinating, and maybe burning and itching around the tip of the penis. Pain and swelling in the testicles are uncommon, but indicate a more serious infection. Rectal and throat infections are possible but uncommon.

Chlamydia Diagnosis

Lab tests for chlamydia are routinely performed on urine from men and swabs from the cervix, vagina, or both from women, and from the throat or rectum if indicated.

Chlamydia Treatment

Chlamydia can be easily cured with antibiotics. A single dose of azithromycin or a week on doxycycline (twice daily) is the best treatment. If allergies are a problem, there are other options available.

All sex partners should be evaluated, tested, and treated, or simply treated as contacts. People with chlamydia should abstain from vaginal or anal intercourse or oral sex until they and their sex partners have completed treatment, otherwise reinfection is possible. Since azithromycin is given in a single dose, you might be tempted to have intercourse right after treatment, but don't. It takes six days for the medicine to work completely, so wait a week before having sex again.

Women whose sex partners haven't been appropriately treated are at a high risk of reinfection. Having multiple infections increases a woman's risk of serious reproductive health complications, including infertility. Retesting should occur three to four months after treatment, especially if a woman doesn't know if her sex partner received treatment. Retesting too soon can yield false positive results, because dead bacteria can hang around for a while and make a test look positive when it's really just picking up dead organisms.

Bacterial Vaginosis: What Is It?

Bacterial vaginosis (BV) is a female condition in which the normal balance of organisms called *lactobacilli* in the vagina is disrupted, and undesirable bacteria grow in larger-than-normal numbers. BV isn't technically an STI, but it's almost never seen in women who've never had sex. The main symptom of BV is a grayish-white, unpleasant-smelling discharge, whose odor is more noticeable after intercourse. Some women might also experience itching or irritation, but that's less common.

It's unclear how women get BV, but some behaviors seem to upset the normal balance of organisms in the vagina and put women at an increased risk of developing BV, including having a new partner, having multiple sex partners, and douching. BV can increase a woman's susceptibility to other STIs, including herpes.

Bacterial Vaginosis Diagnosis

A health care provider gathers secretions from the vagina and looks under the microscope for classic "clue cells"—skin cells covered with bacteria—changes in the vaginal pH, and a lab test that can elicit the fishy odor.

Bacterial Vaginosis Treatment

Although BV sometimes clears up without treatment, most women opt for treatment to deal with the unpleasant symptoms. Also, pregnant women with BV are most often treated to reduce the risk of premature birth. Women with BV who are having a pelvic procedure—an IUD insertion, a pregnancy termination, or upper genital tract surgery—benefit from treatment as well. Treating male partners has no impact on recurrences of BV in women and isn't recommended. The two medicines for BV are metronidazole or clindamycin, which are taken by mouth in pill form or placed in the vagina as creams, gels, or tablets.

NGU: What Is It?

NGU stands for *nongonococcal urethritis*, any infection of the male urethra that is *not* gonorrhea. Chlamydia would fit that description, but there are some infections that men have that aren't gonorrhea or chlamydia but act similarly. There's usually a minimal amount of cloudy discharge from the penis, possibly irritation at the end of the urethra, and often pain with urination. But when testing is done, neither chlamydia nor gonorrhea is present, but there are white cells present on a smear that's been gathered from the end of the penis. Various things can cause NGU: a bacteria called *mycoplasma*, *ureaplasma*, or *trichomoniasis*, and even herpes in the urethra, can show up in this way. We usually don't look specifically for these bugs in the male urethra; we simply treat based on symptoms. NGU is really a syndrome and not a specific germ. The term "NGU" applies to the group of symptoms I described above when combined with pus cells found on a swab from the urethra.

NGU Diagnosis

A definitive diagnosis is made by looking at a slide under a microscope. The slide is prepared from the substance gathered from the end of the penis by the urethral swab. The lab technician stains the slide and looks for the presence of pus cells. If there are urethral discharge and pus cells present but no gonorrhea, then the diagnosis is NGU.

NGU Treatment

NGU is treated exactly like chlamydia, with 1 gram of azithromycin taken all at once or 100 milligrams of doxycycline taken twice daily for a week. Partners should be evaluated and treated as contacts to NGU. If partners aren't treated, the patient will just get NGU again, and the reinfection cycle never stops. And remember, no sex for a week, even if the symptoms disappear.

There can be complications from untreated NGU—involvement of the testicular area, the prostate, and even the joints—so diagnosis and treatment are important for resolving this problem.

SKIN INFESTATIONS

Some conditions are passed from one partner to another and never get inside the body; they just manifest on the skin. But remember that many abnormal skin conditions aren't sexually transmitted, even if they show up in the genital area. For example, lots of men get symptoms of psoriasis on the penis, and it has nothing to do with an STI.

Scabies: What Is It?

Scabies is a skin disease caused by a very small mite. It's common and found worldwide, and it affects people of all races and social classes.

Scabies is spread between sexual partners and in crowded conditions where there's frequent skin-to-skin contact between people, like in households or institutions such as hospitals, child-care facilities, and nursing homes. People can also get scabies may by sharing clothing, towels, and bedding.

Signs of scabies include very itchy, pimple-like skin irritations, burrows, or rashes, especially in the webbing between the fingers and the skin folds on the wrist, elbow, knee, penis, breasts, or shoulder blades. Commonly, there's intense itching that gets worse at night or when showering. Symptoms of scabies can develop within a week or even months after being infected.

Scabies Diagnosis

Scabies is diagnosed most often by a clinician's exam of the burrows or rash. A skin scraping may be taken to look for mites to confirm the diagnosis, but it's difficult to find the mite this way, because it quickly scurries under the skin. So even if a skin scraping or biopsy is taken and no mite is found, it's still possible to have scabies.

Scabies Treatment

Prescription lotions are available to treat scabies and the associated itching. Always follow the directions provided by your clinician, or on the package label or insert. Apply the medication to a clean body from the neck down to the toes. Don't apply the medicine to your eyebrows. Leave the medication on your body for the recommended time, then take a bath or shower to wash it all off. All clothes, bedding, and towels used during the three days before treatment should be washed in hot water and dried in a hot dryer. A second treatment with the same lotion is most often recommended. Pregnant women and children are usually treated with a milder medication.

Anyone who's diagnosed with scabies should have his or her sex partners and household members treated at the same time. Itching may continue for two to three weeks, but that doesn't mean that you still have scabies. Your clinician may prescribe a different medication to relieve itching if it's severe and continuing.

Pubic Lice (Crabs): What Is It?

Pubic lice, nicknamed "crabs," are very small parasitic insects that live in the pubic hair. Crabs can also be found on other body hair, like eyebrows, eyelashes, beard, mustache, chest, and armpits. Pubic lice are different from the head lice that kids get in preschool, which aren't sexually transmitted. Lice move around by crawling; they can't hop or fly.

Pubic lice are most commonly spread by person-to-person sexual contact. Dogs, cats, and other pets don't transmit pubic lice. The main symptom is itching in the pubic hair area.

Pubic Lice Diagnosis

Adult pubic lice are about 1.5 millimeters long and are easily visible with a magnifying glass. An infestation is diagnosed by examining the pubic hair for *nits* (adults) and eggs on the hair shaft or from finding adult crabs in underwear; they appear as little black or brown specks. The nits are cloudy little bundles stuck firmly to the shaft of the pubic hair. Adults are brown and can be picked off the skin. If you put them on a piece of white paper, you can see them move around fairly easily, and that makes the diagnosis simple.

Pubic Lice Treatment

Very effective over-the-counter treatments are available for pubic lice; just read and follow the instructions on the box. Sex partners should be evaluated and treated as needed.

PROTOZOA INFECTIONS

Protozoa cause one sexually transmitted infection: trichomoniasis.

Trichomoniasis: What Is It?

Trichomoniasis is a sexually transmitted infection that affects both women and men, but women are almost always the ones who have symptoms. Often abbreviated as "trich," it's caused by protozoa that swim around in secretions by flapping their "tails," called *flagella*. Trichomoniasis is the most common curable STI in young, sexually active women, and it's estimated that over seven million new cases occur each year in women and men (CDC 2007b).

The vagina and cervix are the most common sites of infection in women, and the urethra is the most common site of infection in men. Trich is sexually transmitted through penis-to-vagina intercourse or vulva-to-vulva contact. Women can acquire the disease from infected men or women, but men usually contract it only from infected women. Trich is rarely seen in men who have sex with men.

Most men with trich don't usually have symptoms, but some men may have an irritation inside the penis, a slight discharge, or a slight burning after urination or ejaculation.

Women who have symptoms of infection often experience a frothy, yellow-green vaginal discharge with a noticeable fishy odor. The infection also may cause discomfort during intercourse and urination, as well as irritation and itching of the genital area. In rare cases, lower abdominal pain can occur. Symptoms usually appear in women within five to twenty-eight days of infection.

Trich Diagnosis

To diagnose trich, a clinician performs a physical examination and laboratory tests. Women are almost always the ones who are diagnosed, whereas men are most often treated as contacts to women who have the infection. In men, trich live in little canals to the sides of the urethra, and are difficult to detect. But in women, trich can be diagnosed by a genital exam, and a microscopic exam or rapid lab test. During the exam, the clinician might note the frothy discharge from the vagina, the fishy odor, or an abnormal looking cervix, commonly called a "strawberry cervix," caused by irritation from the protozoa. Under the microscope, a sample of vaginal secretions will reveal the organism. The microscopic exam is less sensitive than rapid lab tests, but the microscopic exam can be performed within a few minutes in a clinician's office.

Trich Treatment

Trichomoniasis can almost always be cured with metronidazole or tinidazole, and both antibiotics are taken by mouth in a single large dose. An infected man, even a man who has never had symptoms, can continue to infect or reinfect a female partner until he's been treated, so all partners should be treated at the same time to eliminate bouncing trich back and forth. People being treated for trich should avoid sex until they and their sex partners complete treatment and have no symptoms. When mixed with alcohol, metronidazole can make you vomit, so it's best to avoid drinking alcohol for twenty-four hours before or after taking this medication.

Chapter 11

Herpes Resources: Finding What You Need

Recent years have seen the rise of the Internet as a source for all sorts of information. We still get professional journals in our clinic and have a few texts we use for reference, but if we're looking for the latest information on a disease, we jump on the computer first. Though there are some great websites for medical information for the general public, there are also many poor ones that post incorrect, even completely misleading, information. The trick is finding the good ones and knowing whom to believe! Many sites try to sell you products that don't work and that waste your money. Others offer anecdotal experiences as "fact," and others are too biased by personal opinion to be credible. Suffice it to say, if you see something online that sounds too good to be true, it probably is.

I won't try to talk you out of browsing yourself silly when it comes to looking for herpes information on the Net; it's pretty natural to search a lot of sites when you're first diagnosed. However, in this chapter, I'll point you to accurate sources of information. In most cases, I've listed the home page for a website, but most have many more useful pages attached to their home pages. You know the way that goes, right? There are also free telephone hotlines available for patients who want to talk to a person rather than read a website, and I'll list those numbers for you, too.

ACCURATE MEDICAL INFORMATION

Most people search the Web for information about herpes before looking for anything else, like support groups or chat rooms. But it's amazing to me how websites can vary so greatly in the accuracy of their medical content. The sites I list here should agree on most of the basics about genital herpes, but you might occasionally find points where they don't.

CDC: The Centers for Disease Control and Prevention (CDC) is considered by many to be the gold standard for information on accurate approaches to diagnosing, managing, and treating herpes. The general information page on genital herpes is here:

- www.cdc.gov/std/herpes/STDFact-herpes.htm

If you want to see the clinician's "bible" on diagnosing and treating all STIs, you can go to:

- www.cdc.gov/STD/treatment

There you'll find everything you want to know about the history, diagnosis, and treatment of all the STIs commonly found in the United States, and there's an excellent section on genital herpes. This is the resource we use at our clinic to guide our practice in the field of sexual health. You'll find technical specifics like the names and doses of the best medications for a given infection. It also contains information about special circumstances like STIs during pregnancy and in HIV-infected people.

The American Social Health Association (ASHA): ASHA is a non-profit organization that's been around since 1914, and is dedicated to stopping STIs and their serious consequences. The ASHA main page is here:

- www.ashastd.org

At the ASHA website, you can find lots of information about genital herpes by clicking the Herpes Resource Center link. There are links to ongoing clinical trials, personal stories about people with herpes, an online kit with information about testing, the number for the ASHA herpes hotline, locations of support groups, copies of the quarterly publication *The Helper*, and even herpes information in Spanish. You can post messages to a moderated message board to get answers to your questions. You can donate to ASHA if you wish and order products related to herpes or other STIs. There's a page to teach you how to use condoms most effectively and another about how to talk to teenagers about STIs. The website even tells you how you can get involved as a volunteer. ASHA is the best organization around to learn more about STIs and sexual health. Make this and the CDC website your number one online links for herpes information.

Westover Heights Clinic: At my clinic's website, you'll find an approximately twenty-minute-long patient-counseling video that answers many of the questions you may have when you're first diagnosed and addresses issues like, "How did I get this in a monogamous relationship?" and "How will I ever be able to tell future partners I have herpes?" I made the DVD for GlaxoSmithKline, so you can also probably get a copy of it at your clinician's office for free, if you'd like to have it on DVD. You'll also find a free, downloadable copy of *The Updated Herpes Handbook*, a forty-five-page booklet about herpes, if you want to share some basic herpes info with someone else and don't want to part with your own copy of your book. Here's our Web address:

- www.westoverheights.com

The International Herpes Management Forum (IHMF): IHMF is a group devoted to disseminating accurate information about the herpes viruses to clinicians around the world. Here's the Web address:

- www.ihmf.org

IHMF holds an annual medical conference, and the website contains the outcomes of these meetings in the form of monographs, supplemental publications, and guidelines. The website is aimed primarily at professionals, but there are patient resources too, and the motivated learner can understand much of the scientific information. The *Herpes* journal found there is chock-full of heavy-duty scientific research on herpes. It may be too technical for some people, but if you really want to get into Web-based scientific information on herpes and you don't subscribe to Medline, this will give you a lot of what you need.

The American Herpes Foundation (AHF): A more Americanized version of herpes information can be found at the American Herpes Foundation website:

- www.herpes-foundation.org

You'll be surprised by how differently Americans view genital herpes infections from people in other parts of the world. For example, in the United States we test for many more STDs than most European countries, and we're more aggressive about herpes treatment than our European neighbors.

Medline Plus: Another comprehensive educational site is at Medline Plus:

- www.nlm.nih.gov/medlineplus/herpessimplex.html

Here you'll find the basics in both English and Spanish: links to research studies, the latest media releases about herpes, photos, and links for specific populations, like women and teens.

PubMed: If you want to look up a scientific article on a particular topic, visit the PubMed site:

- www.pubmed.com

Anyone can use the site, and you don't have to be a clinician or a scientist. Let's say you want to check out my professional credibility: Should you really believe things I have to say in this book, do I have enough research experience, and have I written credible scientific publications that warrant your confidence? At the top of the page you can search by author. In my case, you'd enter "Warren T herpes," and all the articles by any "Warren T" on genital herpes will be listed. You could also search by topic. Let's say you want to know about herpes vaccines. In the same search space, you would enter "herpes vaccine," and all the articles in the professional literature that address herpes vaccines will be listed. If you enter a topic that may be too broad, like "genital herpes," you'll be drowning in articles, so you've got to be fairly specific. There are directions on the site for how to perform searches, but I find them pretty complicated. Those with more advanced computer skills than I have will probably do just fine. The site posts the very newest articles quickly, so this is the place to get the most up-to-date information. Note: For some articles, you'll only get the abstract, a summary of the research. But for others, you can get the full-text article. After an article has been available for a while, you're more likely to have access to it in its entirety.

HERPES NETWORKING: MESSAGE BOARDS, AND CHAT ROOMS

WebMD: WebMD is an excellent Web resource for current information in all areas of medicine, so it really fits into both the section above and this section. I listed it in this section, because I think one of its most useful offerings is its question-and-answer board on genital herpes. Here's the link:

- www.webmd.com/community/boards

Scroll down to sexual conditions, and choose the genital herpes message board. There's no charge for using the site; you can simply pick a screen name and password, and post a question. Often I'll be the one to answer your question, or another medical professional may post a response, but anyone can participate, including nonmedical folks who have experience with herpes infections. Are you wondering how to have "the talk," for example? Just post your question about it, and a person who's "been there and done that" will likely respond. You couldn't get the name of a specific clinician referral for a particular location, because WebMD doesn't allow that kind of posting, but someone may send you to another link that will get you what you want. There's no limit to the number of questions you can ask, and no questions are too personal or "stupid." The nice thing about posting on the WebMD message board is that it's completely anonymous, so you can feel free to go into details that might be too graphic or uncomfortable for you to ask in person. I also have a blog on WebMD, where I openly speak my mind on sensitive topics. This link will get you there:

- www.blogs.webmd.com/genital-herpes-intimate-conversations

There's another site where you can post concerns about living with herpes on WebMD:

- boards.webmd.com/webx/topics/hd/Sex-and-Relationships/ Genital-Herpes-Living-Day-to-Day

However, you might find it easier to just type "webmd herpes day to day" into your favorite browser.

The Original Herpes Home Page: This well-established site (since 1995) is a great place to do some herpes networking, offering an opportunity to interact online with others who have herpes for information and support:

- www.herpeshomepage.com

Roger, the fellow who runs the website, feels strongly about posting accurate information on his site. He's attended my lectures and takes this herpes-website business very seriously. The "action" on this site is in the well-moderated discussion forums, where a friendly online community and support group has developed. It's a place where a person with herpes can discover that he or she is not alone, and has a shoulder to cry on and a place to vent and learn about the practical aspects of living with the condition. There's even an off-topic forum for chatting about everyday life, exchanging recipes, discussing books, or asking about home repairs. There's no medical professional who answers questions at this site, nor is one needed. "Newbies" will find a warm welcome here as they adjust to having herpes.

MedHelp: If you decide to become more familiar with STIs, you'll start to recognize the names Dr. Edward Hook and Dr. Hunter Handsfield. They've been leaders in the field for many years. You can write a question to Edward or Hunter at their MedHelp website:

- www.medhelp.org/forums/STD/wwwboard.html

There's a fee for posting at this "expert" site. However, MedHelp also offers a free site for just talking with others about herpes:

- www.medhelp.org/forums/show/195.

The American Social Health Association (www.ashastd.org), which we talked about earlier, also has message boards available. Here's the link:

- www.ashastd.org/phpbb/index.php

ONLINE DATING

We all know about online dating, and some of us have even tried it. But did you know that there are several online dating services especially for people with STIs like genital herpes? One of the largest of these is at Antopia:

- www.MPwH.com (stands for "Meet People with Herpes")

I personally don't believe that people with herpes should limit themselves to only dating others with herpes, but I think herpes dating services offer a place for newly diagnosed people to "put a toe in the water." Are you terrified of having "the talk"? This website and others like it allow you to skip that step. Registered users (and you don't have to use your real name) indicate their STI status when they sign up so that "all the cards are on the table." You can search by city, state, STI status, age, and so on. Your contact information can be as private as you'd like (and it should be). There's a fee to subscribe, and you may want to eventually move beyond needing such sites to meet people. In fact, I hope you do. But I see such sites as one resource. Think of it this way: Let's say you have a standard poodle, and you just love that breed—you show it, you train it, and you just think it's terrific. If you're looking to date people, you might see if there's a group of standard-poodle lovers like yourself, who share your particular interest. For example, Jewish singles often try JDate, because they can find others who have similar religious beliefs. There are singles sites for just about every area of interest. You may decide that you can *only* date people with herpes (which I think is a big mistake), but sites like this can provide a start. Of course, all the usual precautions involved in any kind of Internet meeting or dating should be followed when using such sites. There are many wonderful people out there surfing for friendship and love, but there are "sickos" and criminals too. Keep your guard up and use these sites wisely.

DIAGNOSING HERPES

Herpes Diagnosis is a site developed by the clinicians at the University of Washington:

- www.herpesdiagnosis.com

These people know more about herpes than, well, just about anyone. If you want to know about the latest tests for herpes and how to interpret them, this is the place to go. Is your clinician behind the times in knowledge about herpes testing? You can direct your clinician here or print selected pages from this site to give to him or her. America's herpes diagnosis "guru," Rhoda Ashley-Morrow, Ph.D., is one of the forces behind this site, and when her hand is on the steering wheel, you can have confidence in the direction you're going in.

If you want to get a confirmatory Western blot test done at the University of Washington, go to the UW Clinical Virology Laboratory site:

- http://depts.washington.edu/rspvirus/herpes.htm

It provides information to your clinician on how to draw, prepare, and ship the blood sample for testing.

Did your clinician do the correct test? Is he or she even willing to do it? Have you run into a brick wall over a type-specific IgG blood antibody test, for example? There are websites where you can order your own test, such as at HealthCheckUSA:

- www.healthcheckusa.com

Indicate your town, state, and the test you want, and the order can be managed entirely online. You'll receive the proper paperwork to get your blood drawn at a convenient location, and receive your results by e-mail. For an extra fee, a physician will interpret the results for you. These sites don't normally bill your insurance company, but they do accept credit cards. Online testing leaves much to be desired; the face-to-face contact of an office visit with good counseling is much better. But the reality of herpes testing is that some clinicians don't know which tests to order, give poor information about the test results they get, and aren't even aware that antibody tests can identify specific herpes types! Some even refuse to order testing, because they wouldn't know how to interpret the results. This service can help you if you need to go beyond your current clinician's knowledge level regarding herpes and take your diagnosis into your own hands.

RESEARCH STUDIES

Are you interested in participating in a study about genital herpes? Check out the site at CenterWatch:

- www.centerwatch.com

Here you can find a list of clinical research trials for various health conditions. You can set yourself up to be notified of trials for medications and treatments for a particular condition, as well as learn more about the clinical trial process.

Here's another site you might like to check out:

- http://clinicaltrials.gov

PATIENT MEDICINE ASSISTANCE

Are you having difficulty paying for your antiviral medication? Remember that both acyclovir and famciclovir are available as generics. However, most pharmaceutical companies that still have drugs on patent will offer patients with restricted access (lack of money or insurance) a way to get their drugs. As of this writing, Valtrex is the only herpes medication that's still under patent. And at the Valtrex website, you can find a program that offers varying degrees of help for acquiring the drug:

- www.valtrex.com

There are downloadable coupons for discounts when filling your prescriptions. If your income is somewhat limited or you don't have prescription insurance coverage, programs are available to help pay for the medicine. For those on a severely limited income, there are programs that provide medicine for only a few dollars a year, if you work with your clinician or pharmacist to enroll. If you qualify, don't hesitate to use these programs; they exist for people in need and should be used for that purpose.

THE NEXT BIG THING

For information on the latest treatments and vaccines in early stages of development, you might wish to visit the following sites. These companies are all working on herpes vaccines or treatment, and they're probably just the tip of the iceberg:

- Astellas Pharma   www.astellas.com
- Genocea Biosciences   www.genocea.com
- Antigenics   www.antigenics.com

SUPPORT HOTLINES

Have an urgent question that needs an answer *now*? There are two hotlines that you can call for accurate herpes information. As with the websites, there can be some variation in the information that patients receive, but overall, these are wonderful, free resources for folks with STI questions.

One is operated by ASHA as part of the Herpes Resource Center, which we talked about earlier. The hotline, which receives over 180,000 calls a year, provides accurate information and referrals to people concerned about herpes. Here's the phone number:

- 1-800-227-8922

It's available from 9:00 a.m. to 8:00 p.m., Monday through Friday, eastern time. The hotline is supported by donations from individuals like you, foundations, and businesses. Sometimes there can be quite a wait, but hang in there.

Another hotline is the one provided by the CDC. It's available seven days a week, twenty-four hours a day, and you can speak to someone in Spanish or English. Here's the phone number:

- 1-800-CDC-INFO (1-800-232-4636)

They can answer your questions and refer you to STI services in your area.

So as you can see, if you're seeking information about genital herpes, there's no shortage of excellent places to get it. Again, choose your resources carefully, and beware of anything that sounds too good to be true. You might be a little vulnerable right now to anything that offers you hope for a much better life with herpes. The websites and phone numbers listed in this chapter have been carefully evaluated and will serve your needs with accuracy and kindness.

Reference List

Abu-Raddad, L. J., A. S. Magaret, C. Celum, A. Wald, I. M. Longini, Jr., S. G. Self, and L. Corey. 2008. Genital herpes has played a more important role than any other sexually transmitted infection in driving HIV prevalence in Africa. *PLoS ONE* 3(5):e2230.

American College of Obstetricians and Gynecologists (ACOG). 1999. Management of herpes in pregnancy. Practice bulletin 8 (October):NGC:003096.

Aoki, F. Y., S. Tyring, F. Diaz-Mitoma, G. Gross, J. Gao, and K. Hamed. 2006. Single-day, patient-initiated famciclovir therapy for recurrent genital herpes: A randomized, double-blind, placebo-controlled trial. *Clinical Infectious Diseases* 42 (1):8–13.

Ashley-Morrow, R., E. Krantz, and A. Wald. 2003. Time course of sero-conversion by HerpesSelect ELISA after acquisition of genital herpes simplex virus type 1 (HSV-1) or HSV-2. *Sexually Transmitted Diseases* 30 (4):310–14.

Bavaro, J. B., L. Drolette, D. M. Koelle, J. Almekinder, T. Warren, S. Tyring, and A. Wald. 2008. One-day regimen of valacyclovir for treatment of recurrent genital herpes simplex virus 2 infection. *Sexually Transmitted Diseases* 35 (4):383–86.

Benedetti, J., L. Corey, and R. Ashley. 1994. Recurrence rates in genital herpes after symptomatic first-episode infection. *Annals of Internal Medicine* 121 (11):847–54.

Bodsworth, N. J., R. J. Crooks, S. Borelli, G. Vejlsgaard, J. Paavonen, A. M. Worm, N. Uexkull, J. Esmann, A. Strand, A. J. Ingamells, and

A. Gibb. 1997. Valaciclovir versus aciclovir in patient initiated treatment of recurrent genital herpes: A randomised, double blind clinical trial—International Valaciclovir HSV Study Group. *Genitourinary Medicine* 73 (2):110–16.

Brown, Z. A., J. Benedetti, R. Ashley, S. Burchett, S. Selke, S. Berry, L. A. Vontver, and L. Corey. 1991. Neonatal herpes simplex virus infection in relation to asymptomatic maternal infection at the time of labor. *New England Journal of Medicine* 324 (18):1247–52.

Brown, Z. A., S. Selke, J. Zeh, J. Kopelman, A. Maslow, R. L. Ashley, D. H. Watts, S. Berry, M. Herd, and L. Corey. 1997. The acquisition of herpes simplex virus during pregnancy. *New England Journal of Medicine* 337 (8):509–15.

Brown, Z. A., A. Wald, R. A. Morrow, S. Selke, J. Zeh, and L. Corey. 2003. Effect of serologic status and cesarean delivery on transmission rates of herpes simplex virus from mother to infant. *Journal of the American Medical Association* 289 (2):203–09.

Bryson, Y., M. Dillon, D. I. Bernstein, J. Radolf, P. Zakowski, and E. Garratty. 1993. Risk of acquisition of genital herpes simplex virus type 2 in sex partners of persons with genital herpes: A prospective couple study. *Journal of Infectious Diseases* 167 (4):942–46.

Celum, C., A. Wald, J. Hughes, J. Sanchez, S. Reid, S. Delany-Moretlwe, F. Cowan, M. Casapia, A. Ortiz, J. Fuchs, S. Buchbinder, B. Koblin, S. Zwerski, S. Rose, J. Wang, and L. Corey—HPTN 039 Protocol Team. 2008. Effect of acyclovir on HIV-1 acquisition in herpes simplex virus 2 seropositive women and men who have sex with men: A randomised, double-blind, placebo-controlled trial. *Lancet* 371 (9630):2109–19.

Centers for Disease Control and Prevention (CDC). 1998. Recommendations for prevention and control of hepatitis C virus (HCV) infection and HCV-related chronic disease. MMWR Recommendations and Reports 47 (RR19):1–39.

———. 2000. Tracking the hidden epidemics: Trends in STDs in the United States 2000:1–31. http://www.cdc.gov/std/Trends2000/Trends2000.pdf. Accessed October 2008.

————. 2006. Sexually transmitted diseases: Treatment guidelines 2006. http://www.cdc.gov/std/treatment/default.htm. Accessed June 2008.

————. 2007a. Sexually transmitted diseases: Chlamydia—CDC fact sheet. http://www.cdc.gov/std/chlamydia/STDFact-Chlamydia. htm#symptoms. Accessed June 2008.

————. 2007b. Sexually transmitted diseases: Trichomoniasis—CDC fact sheet. http://www.cdc.gov/std/trichomonas/STDFact-Trichomoniasis. htm#Common. Accessed June 2008.

Cherpes, T. L., M. A. Melan, J. A. Kant, L. A. Cosentino, L. A. Meyn, and S. L. Hillier. 2005. Genital tract shedding of herpes simplex virus type 2 in women: Effects of hormonal contraception, bacterial vaginosis, and vaginal group B Streptococcus colonization. *Clinical Infectious Diseases* 40 (10):1422–28.

Cohen, F., M. E. Kemeny, K. A. Kearney, L. S. Zegans, J. M. Neuhaus, and M. A. Conant. 1999. Persistent stress as a predictor of genital herpes recurrence. *Archives of Internal Medicine* 159 (20):2430–36.

Corey, L. 1988. First-episode, recurrent, and asymptomatic herpes simplex infections. *Journal of the American Academy of Dermatology* 18 (1, pt. 2):169–72.

Corey, L., A. Wald, R. Patel, S. L. Sacks, S. K. Tyring, T. Warren, J. M. Douglas, Jr., J. Paavonen, R. A. Morrow, K. R. Beutner, L. S. Stratchounsky, G. Mertz, O. N. Keene, H. A. Watson, D. Tait, M. Vargas-Cortes for the Valacyclovir HSV Transmission Study Group. 2004. Once-daily valacyclovir to reduce the risk of transmission of genital herpes. *New England Journal of Medicine* 350 (1):11–20.

Danve-Szatanek, C., M. Aymard, D. Thouvenot, F. Morfin, G. Agius, I. Bertin, S. Billaudel, B. Chanzy, M. Coste-Burel, L. Finkielsztejn, H. Fleury, T. Hadou, C. Henquell, H. Lafeuille, M. E. Lafon, A. Le Faou, M. C. Legrand, L. Maille, C. Mengelle, P. Morand, F. Morinet, E. Nicand, S. Omar, B. Picard, B. Pozzetto, J. Puel, D. Raoult, C. Scieux, M. Segondy, J. M. Seigneurin, R. Teyssou, and C. Zandotti. 2004. Surveillance network for herpes simplex virus resistance to antiviral drugs: 3-year follow-up. *Journal of Clinical Microbiology* 42 (1):242–49.

Engelberg R., D. Carrell, E. Krantz, L. Corey, and A. Wald. 2003. Natural history of genital herpes simplex virus type 1 infection. *Sexually Transmitted Diseases* 30 (2):174–77.

Fife, K. H., R. A. Barbarash, T. Rudolph, B. Degregorio, and R. Roth. 1997. Valaciclovir versus acyclovir in the treatment of first-episode genital herpes infection: Results of an international, multicenter, double-blind, randomized clinical trial—The Valaciclovir International Herpes Simplex Virus Study Group. *Sexually Transmitted Diseases* 24 (8):481–86.

Fife, K. H., T. J. Warren, S. E. Justus, and C. K. Heitman. 2008. An international, randomized, double-blind, placebo-controlled study of valacyclovir for the suppression of herpes simplex virus type 2 genital herpes in newly diagnosed patients. *Sexually Transmitted Diseases* 35 (7):668–73.

Freeman, E. E., H. A. Weiss, J. R. Glynn, P. L. Cross, J. A. Whitworth, and R. J. Hayes. 2006. Herpes simplex virus 2 infection increases HIV acquisition in men and women: Systematic review and meta-analysis of longitudinal studies. *AIDS* 20 (1):73–83.

FUTURE II Study Group. 2007. Quadrivalent vaccine against human papillomavirus to prevent high-grade cervical lesions. *New England Journal of Medicine* 356 (19):1915–27.

Gardella, C., and Z. A. Brown. 2007. Managing genital herpes infections in pregnancy. *Cleveland Clinic Journal of Medicine* 74 (3):217–24.

Gilbert, L., K. Scanlon, R. Peterson, and C. Ebel. 2005. Patient and partner perceptions about preventing genital herpes transmission. *Herpes* 12 (3):60–65.

Gilbert, S. C. 2007. Management and prevention of recurrent herpes labialis in immunocompetent patients. *Herpes* 14 (3):56–61.

Gnann, Jr., J. W., and R. J. Whitley. 2002. Clinical practice: Herpes zoster. *New England Journal of Medicine* 347 (5):340–46.

Golden, M. R., R. Ashley-Morrow, P. Swenson, W. R. Hogrefe, H. H. Handsfield, and A. Wald. 2005. Herpes simplex virus type 2 (HSV-2) Western blot confirmatory testing among men testing positive for HSV-2 using the focus enzyme-linked immunosorbent assay in a sexually transmitted disease clinic. *Sexually Transmitted Diseases* 32 (12):771–77.

Gupta, R., A. Wald, E. Krantz, S. Selke, T. Warren, M. Vargas-Cortes, G. Miller, and L. Corey. 2004. Valacyclovir and acyclovir for suppression of shedding of herpes simplex virus in the genital tract. *Journal of Infectious Diseases* 190 (8):1374–81.

Gupta, R., T. Warren, and A. Wald. 2007. Genital herpes. Lancet 370 (9605):2127–37.

Handsfield, H. H., T. Warren, M. Werner, and J. A. Phillips. 2007. Suppressive therapy with valacyclovir in early genital herpes: A pilot study of clinical efficacy and herpes-related quality of life. *Sexually Transmitted Diseases* 34(6):339-43.

Hollier, L. M., and G. D. Wendel. 2008. Third trimester antiviral prophylaxis for preventing maternal genital herpes simplex virus (HSV) recurrences and neonatal infection. *Cochrane Database of Systematic Reviews*, issue 1 (January 23), art. no.: CD004946, doi: 10.1002/14651858.CD004946.pub2.

Hu, D., and S. Goldie. 2008. The economic burden of noncervical human papillomavirus disease in the United States. *American Journal of Obstetrics and Gynecology* 198 (5):500.e1-7.

Kerkering, K., C. Gardella, S. Selke, E. Krantz, L. Corey, and A. Wald. 2006. Isolation of herpes simplex virus from the genital tract during symptomatic recurrence on the buttocks. *Obstetrics and Gynecology* 108 (4):947–52.

Kinghorn, G. 2002. Debate: The argument for—Should all pregnant women be offered type-specific serological screening for HSV infection? *Herpes* 9 (2):46–7.

Lafferty W. E., R. W. Coombs, J. Benedetti, C. Critchlow, and L. Corey. 1987. Recurrences after oral and genital herpes simplex virus infection: Influence of site of infection and viral type. *New England Journal of Medicine* 316 (23):1444–49.

Langenberg, A. G. M., L. Corey, R. L. Ashley, W. P. Leong, and S. E. Straus for the Chiron HSV Vaccine Study Group. 1999. A prospective study of new infections with herpes simplex virus type 1 and type 2. *New England Journal of Medicine* 341 (19):1432–38.

Leone, P., D. T. Fleming, A. W. Gilsenan, L. Li, and S. Justus. 2004. Seroprevalence of herpes simplex virus-2 in suburban primary care offices in the United States. *Sexually Transmitted Diseases* 31 (5):311–16.

Looker, K. J., and G. P. Garnett. 2005. A systematic review of the epidemiology and interaction of herpes simplex virus types 1 and 2. *Sexually Transmitted Infections* 81 (2):103–07.

Malkin, J. E. 2004. Epidemiology of genital herpes simplex virus infection in developed countries. *Herpes* 11 (Suppl 1):2A–23A.

Mark, K. E., L. Corey, T. C. Meng, A. S. Magaret, M. L. Huang, S. Selke, H. B. Slade, S. K. Tyring, T. Warren, S. L. Sacks, P. Leone, V. A. Bergland, and A. Wald. 2007. Topical resiquimod 0.01% gel decreases herpes simplex virus type 2 genital shedding: A randomized, controlled trial. *Journal of Infectious Diseases* 195 (9):1324–31.

Mark, K. E., A. Wald, A. S. Magaret, S. Selke, L. Olin, M. L. Huang, and L. Corey. 2008. Rapidly cleared episodes of herpes simplex virus reactivation in immunocompetent adults. *Journal of Infectious Diseases* 198 (8):1141–49.

McLarnon, L. D., and D. G. Kaloupek. 1988. Psychological investigation of genital herpes recurrence: Prospective assessment and cognitive-behavioral intervention for a chronic physical disorder. *Health Psychology* 7 (3):231–49.

Mertz, G. J., J. Benedetti, R. Ashley, S. A. Selke, and L. Corey. 1992. Risk factors for the sexual transmission of genital herpes. *Annals of Internal Medicine* 116 (3):197–202.

Miller, C. S., and R. J. Danaher. 2008. Asymptomatic shedding of herpes simplex virus (HSV) in the oral cavity. *Oral Surgery, Oral Medicine, Oral Pathology, Oral Radiology, and Endodontics* 105(1):43–50.

Mindel, A. 1996. Psychological and psychosexual implications of herpes simplex virus infections. *Scandinavian Journal of Infectious Diseases Supplement* 100:27–32.

Miyai, T., K. R. Turner, C. K. Kent, and J. Klausner. 2004. The psychosocial impact of testing individuals with no history of genital herpes for herpes simplex virus type 2. *Sexually Transmitted Diseases* 31 (9):517–21.

Mohllajee, A. P., K. M. Curtis, S. L. Martins, and H. B. Peterson. 2006. Hormonal contraceptive use and risk of sexually transmitted infections: A systematic review. *Contraception* 73 (2):154–65.

Nagot, N., A. Ouedraogo, I. Konate, H. A. Weiss, V. Foulongne, M. C. Defer, A. Sanon, P. Becquart, M. Segondy, A. Sawadogo, P. van de Perre, and P. Mayaud—ANRS 1285 Study Group. 2008. Roles of clinical and subclinical reactivated herpes simplex virus type 2 infection and human immunodeficiency virus type 1 (HIV-1)-induced immunosuppression on genital and plasma HIV-1 levels. *Journal of Infectious Diseases* 198 (2):241–49.

Nahass, G. T., B. A. Goldstein, W. Y. Zhu, U. Serfling, N. S. Penneys, and C. L. Leonardi. 1992. Comparison of Tzanck smear, viral culture, and DNA diagnostic methods in detection of herpes simplex and varicella-zoster infection. *Journal of the American Medical Association* 268 (18):2541–44.

Paavonen, J., D. Jenkins, F. X. Bosch, P. Naud, J. Salmerón, C. M. Wheeler, S. N. Chow, D. L. Apter, H. C. Kitchener, X. Castellsague, N. S. de Carvalho, S. R. Skinner, D. M. Harper, J. A. Hedrick, U. Jaisamrarn, G. A. Limson, M. Dionne, W. Quint, B. Spiessens, P. Peeters, F. Struyf, S. L. Wieting, M. O. Lehtinen, and G. Dubin—HPV PATRICIA study group. 2007. Efficacy of a prophylactic adjuvanted bivalent L1 virus-like-particle vaccine against infection with human papillomavirus types 16 and 18 in young women: An interim analysis of a phase III double-blind, randomised controlled trial. *Lancet* 369 (9580):2161–70.

Plummer, M., M. Schiffman, P. E. Castle, D. Maucort-Boulch, and C. M. Wheeler for the ALTS Group. 2007. A 2-year prospective study of human papillomavirus persistence among women with a cytological diagnosis of atypical squamous cells of undetermined significance or low-grade squamous intraepithelial lesion. *Journal of Infectious Diseases* 195 (11):1582–89.

Posavad, C. M., A. Wald, N. Hosken, M. L. Huang, D. M. Koelle, R. L. Ashley, and L. Corey. 2003. T cell immunity to herpes simplex viruses in seronegative subjects: Silent infection or acquired immunity? *Journal of Immunology* 170 (8):4380–88.

Rand, K. H., E. F. Hoon, J. K. Massey, and J. H. Johnson. 1990. Daily stress and recurrence of genital herpes simplex. *Archives of Internal Medicine* 150 (9):1889–93.

Rein, M. 2000. Stress and genital herpes recurrences in women. *Journal of the American Medical Association* 283 (11):1394.

Reitano, M., S. Tyring, W. Lang, C. Thoming, A. M. Worm, S. Borelli, L. O. Chambers, J. M. Robinson, and L. Corey. 1998. Valaciclovir for the suppression of recurrent genital herpes simplex virus infection: A large-scale dose range-finding study—International Valaciclovir HSV Study Group. *Journal of Infectious Diseases* 178 (3):603–10.

Roberts, C. M., J. R. Pfister, and S. J. Spear. 2003. Increasing proportion of herpes simplex virus type 1 as a cause of genital herpes infection in college students. *Sexually Transmitted Diseases* 30 (10):797–800.

Rosenthal, S. L., G. D. Zimet, J. S. Leichliter, L. R. Stanberry, K. H. Fife, W. Tu, and D. I. Bernstein. 2006. The psychosocial impact of serological diagnosis of asymptomatic herpes simplex virus type 2 infection. *Sexually Transmitted Infections* 82 (2):154–57; discussion 157–58.

Sacks, S. L., P. D. Griffiths, L. Corey, C. Cohen, A. Cunningham, G. M. Dusheiko, S. Self, S. Spruance, L. R. Stanberry, A. Wald, and R. J. Whitley. 2004. HSV shedding. *Antiviral Research* 63 (Suppl. 1):S19–26.

Schacker, T. 2001. The role of HSV in the transmission and progression of HIV. *Herpes* 8 (2):46–49.

Sheffield, J. S., D. N. Fish, L. M. Hollier, S. Cadematori, B. J. Nobles, and G. D. Wendel, Jr. 2002. Acyclovir concentrations in human breast milk after valaciclovir administration. *American Journal of Obstetrics and Gynecology* 186 (1):100–02.

Sheffield, J. S., J. B. Hill, L. M. Hollier, V. R. Laibl, S. W. Roberts, P. J. Sanchez, and G. D. Wendel, Jr. 2006. Valacyclovir prophylaxis to prevent recurrent herpes at delivery: A randomized clinical trial. *Obstetrics and Gynecology* 108 (1):695.

Sheffield, J. S., L. M. Hollier, J. B. Hill, G. S. Stuart, and G. D. Wendel. 2003. Acyclovir prophylaxis to prevent herpes simplex virus recurrence at delivery: A systematic review. Obstetrics and Gynecology 102 (6):1396–1403.

Soriano V., A. Mocroft, J. Rockstroh, B. Ledergerber, B. Knysz, S. Chaplinskas, L. Peters, A. Karlsson, C. Katlama, C. Toro, B. Kupfer, M. Vogel, and J. Lundgren for the EuroSIDA Study Group. 2008. Spontaneous viral clearance, viral load, and genotype distribution of hepatitis C virus (HCV) in HIV-infected patients with anti-HCV antibodies in Europe. *Journal of Infectious Diseases* 198 (September 3), doi:10.1086/592171, http://www.journals.uchicago.edu/doi/full/10.1086/592171. Accessed June 2008.

Stanberry, L. R., S. L. Spruance, A. L. Cunningham, D. I. Bernstein, A. Mindel, S. Sacks, S. Tyring, F. Y. Aoki, M. Slaoui, M. Denis, P. Vandepapeliere, G. Dubin—GlaxoSmithKline Herpes Vaccine Efficacy Study Group. 2002. Glycoprotein-D-adjuvant vaccine to prevent genital herpes. *New England Journal of Medicine* 347 (21):1652–61.

Stone, K. M., R. Reiff-Eldridge, A. D. White, J. F. Cordero, Z. Brown, E. Russell Alexander, and E. B. Andrews. 2004. Pregnancy outcomes following systemic prenatal acyclovir exposure: Conclusions from the International Acyclovir Pregnancy Registry, 1984–1999. *Birth Defects Research: Clinical and Molecular Teratology* 70 (4):201–07.

Tyring, S. K., D. Baker, and W. Snowden. 2002. Valacyclovir for herpes simplex virus infection: Long-term safety and sustained efficacy after 20 years' experience with acyclovir. *Journal of Infectious Diseases* 186 (Suppl. 1):S40–46.

U.S. Preventive Services Task Force. 2001. Screening for chlamydial infection: Recommendations and rationale. *American Journal of Preventive Medicine* 20 (Suppl. 3):90–94.

Wald, A., D. Carrell, M. Remington, E. Kexel, J. Zeh, and L. Corey. 2002. Two-day regimen of acyclovir for treatment of recurrent genital herpes simplex virus type 2 infection. *Clinical Infectious Diseases* 34 (7):944–48.

Wald, A., M. L. Huang, D. Carrell, S. Selke, and L. Corey. 2003. Polymerase chain reaction for detection of herpes simplex virus (HSV) DNA on mucosal surfaces: Comparison with HSV isolation in cell culture. *Journal of Infectious Diseases* 188 (9):1345–51.

Wald, A., E. Krantz, S. Selke, E. Lairson, R. A. Morrow, and J. Zeh. 2006a. Knowledge of partners' genital herpes protects against herpes simplex virus type 2 acquisition. *Journal of Infectious Diseases* 194 (1):42–52.

Wald, A., A. G. M. Langenberg, E. Krantz, J. M. Douglas, Jr., H. H. Handsfield, R. P. DiCarlo, A. A. Adimora, A. E. Izu, R. A. Morrow, and L. Corey. 2005. The relationship between condom use and herpes simplex virus acquisition. *Annals of Internal Medicine* 143 (10):707–13.

Wald, A., A. G. M. Langenberg, K. Link, A. E. Izu, R. Ashley, T. Warren, S. Tyring, J. M. Douglas, Jr., and L. Corey. 2001. Effect of condoms on reducing the transmission of herpes simplex virus type 2 from men to women. *Journal of the American Medical Association* 285 (24):3100–06.

Wald, A., S. Selke, T. Warren, F. Y. Aoki, S. Sacks, F. Diaz-Mitoma, and L. Corey. 2006b. Comparative efficacy of famciclovir and valacyclovir for suppression of recurrent genital herpes and viral shedding. *Sexually Transmitted Diseases* 33 (9):529–33.

Wald, A., J. Zeh, S. Selke, T. Warren, A. J. Ryncarz, R. Ashley, J. N. Krieger, and L. Corey. 2000. Reactivation of genital herpes simplex virus type 2 infection in asymptomatic seropositive persons. *New England Journal of Medicine* 342 (12):844–50.

Whitley, R., E. A. Davis, and N. Suppapanya. 2007. Incidence of neonatal herpes simplex virus infections in a managed-care population. *Sexually Transmitted Diseases* 34 (9):704–08.

Wright, T. C., F. X. Bosch, E. L. Franco, J. Cuzick, J. T. Schiller, G. P. Garnett, and A. Meheus. 2006. Chapter 30: HPV vaccines and screening in the prevention of cervical cancer; conclusions from a 2006 workshop of international experts. *Vaccine* 24 (Suppl. 3):S251–61.

Xu, F., L. E. Markowitz, S. L. Gottlieb, and S. M. Berman. 2007. Seroprevalence of herpes simplex virus types 1 and 2 in pregnant women in the United States. *American Journal of Obstetrics and Gynecology* 196 (1):43.e1–6.

Xu, F., M. R. Sternberg, B. J. Kottiri, G. M. McQuillan, F. K. Lee, A. J. Nahmias, S. M. Berman, and L. E. Markowitz. 2006. Trends in herpes simplex virus type 1 and type 2 seroprevalence in the United States. *Journal of the American Medical Association* 296 (8):964–73.

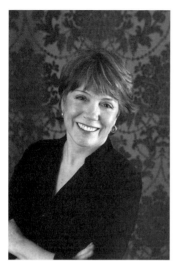

Alyssa Jul Photography

Terri Warren, RN, NP, has owned and operated Westover Heights Clinic in Portland, OR, a private clinic specializing in sexually transmitted diseases, for more than twenty-five years. She speaks nationally and internationally on the topic of genital herpes and has authored papers published in several medical journals. An accomplished researcher, Warren has been the investigator or subinvestigator in more than eighty clinical trials, most of which involved genital herpes infections. She is also the herpes expert on WebMD.com, where she answers readers' questions about genital herpes infections. Warren is author of *The Updated Herpes Handbook* and coauthor of *Tender Talk*.

Index

disclosing your herpes, 107-131; contents of "the talk" for, 118-120; to current partners, 122-125; to employers and coworkers, 126-127; to family members, 126; to friends, 126; to health care providers, 127; natural opportunities for, 116-117; possible responses to, 120-122; to potential partners, 107-122; to previous partners, 125-126; questions and answers about, 129-131; reasons for, 107-113; setting for, 118; style of "the talk" for, 117-118; timing considerations for, 115; trust and intimacy issues in, 114-115

doxycycline, 172, 174

drying agents, 99

E

Elion, Gertrude, 84

ELISA test, 55-56, 64, 66

embarrassment, 138-139

emotional reactions: anger, 135-136; confusion, 137; decreased self-esteem, 145; depression, 142-144; embarrassment, 138-139; fear, 137-138; guilt, 136; immediate reactions, 134-139; isolation, 141-142; loss, 139-140; relief, 144; rethinking, 145-150; shame, 141; shock/surprise, 134; stigma, 140; sustained reactions, 134-139. *See also* psychological responses to herpes

employers, disclosing your herpes to, 126-127

episodic suppression, 92-93

episodic therapy, 91-92

Epstein-Barr virus (EBV), 14

equivocal results, 56

Express test, 56-57

eyes, herpes of, 20

F

false positive/negative, 48

famciclovir (Famvir), 85, 86, 88, 91

family members, disclosing your herpes to, 126

fear, 137-138

feelings. *See* emotional reactions

fever blisters. *See* cold sores

first-outbreak treatment, 86-87

flagella, 177

friends, disclosing your herpes to, 126

G

Gardasil vaccine, 164

genital herpes: breastfeeding and, 77; childbirth and, 71-72; diagnosis of, 8-9, 45-67; disclosing to others, 107-131; HIV and, 60, 157-160; information resources on, 179-189; outbreak triggers for, 27; pregnancy and, 70-78; prevalence of, 1, 21; psychological responses to, 133-155; symptoms of, 23-25; tests for, 8-9; transmission of, 5-6, 7, 31-44; treatments for,

7, 8, 83-105; viruses associated with, 12-13, 20-21, 23-26; women's issues related to, 68-81. *See also* herpes viruses
genital shedding, 28
genital sores, 59
genital warts, 162-163
glycoprotein G specific (gG-based) tests, 54
gonorrhea, 170-171
Gram's stain, 170
guilt, 136

H

Handsfield, Hunter, 184
health care providers: disclosing your herpes to, 127; intentional misdiagnosis by, 17
HealthCheckUSA, 186
helicase-primase inhibitors, 96
hepatitis B virus, 166-167
hepatitis C virus, 165-166
Herpes Diagnosis website, 186
Herpes Home Page website, 184
herpes keratitis, 20
herpes simplex virus type 1 (HSV 1), 6, 12-13, 19-21; common questions about, 29-30; diseases caused by, 19-21; genital herpes and, 20-21; location of, 19, 20, 28; oral outbreak triggers for, 21; prevalence of, 21; shedding associated with, 19-20, 28; transmission of, 34-35
herpes simplex virus type 2 (HSV 2), 6-7, 13, 22-28; characteristics of, 25-26;

common questions about, 29-30; demographics of, 22-23; diseases caused by, 23-26; genital herpes and, 23-26; location of, 26-27, 28; outbreak triggers for, 27; prevalence of, 22-23, 27-28; shedding associated with, 28; transmission of, 34-35; vaccine for, 100
herpes support groups, 155
herpes viruses, 12-30; cytomegalovirus, 14; Epstein-Barr, 14; herpes simplex virus type 1, 6, 12-13, 19-21, 28; herpes simplex virus type 2, 6-7, 13, 22-28; human herpes virus 6, 14-15; human herpes virus 7, 15; human herpes virus 8, 15; varicella-zoster, 13, 15-19. *See also* genital herpes
herpes zoster, 13, 16
HerpeSelect tests, 55-57, 63
HIV and herpes, 60, 157-160; CD4 T cells and, 158-159; experimental treatment for, 159-160; viral shedding and, 158
homeopathic treatments, 102-103
Hook, Edward, 184
hotlines, support, 188-189
HPV. *See* human papillomavirus
human herpes virus 6 (HHV 6), 14-15
human herpes virus 7 (HHV 7), 15
human herpes virus 8 (HHV 8), 15

human papillomavirus (HPV), 162-165; cervical cancer and, 7, 78-79, 163, 164; diagnosis of, 80, 163; genital warts and, 162-163; treatments for, 163-164; vaccine for, 164-165

Hutchings, George, 84

I

ice treatment, 99

IgG antibody tests, 9, 54, 58

IgM antibody tests, 54, 58

imiquimod (Aldara), 95, 163, 168

immune-modulator drugs, 95-96

Immunoblot test, 56

index values, 55

information resources, 179-189; diagnosing herpes, 186-187; latest treatments, 188; medical information, 180-183; medication assistance, 187-188; networking websites, 183-185; online dating, 185; research studies, 187; support hotlines, 188-189

International Herpes Management Forum (IHMF), 181

Internet: diagnostic tests via, 186-187; herpes treatments sold on, 97, 103; medical information on, 180-183; networking sites on, 183-185; online dating via, 185; patient medicine assistance via, 187-188; reliability of info found on, 179; research studies on, 187

isolation, 141-142

K

Kaposi's sarcoma, 15

L

lab tests, 48-60; blood antibody tests, 52-60; questions for clinicians about, 60-62; virus swab tests, 48-52

labor precautions/procedures, 71-72

lactobacilli, 172

LEEP procedure, 164

legal issues, 112

loose clothing, 99

loss, feelings of, 139-140

lysine, 97

M

marriage. *See* relationships

MedHelp website, 184

medical information resources, 180-183

medications: antiviral vs. antibiotic, 83-85; episodic suppression, 92-93; first-outbreak, 86-87; immune-modulator, 95-96; outbreak therapy, 91-92; questions and answers about, 100-105; resistance to, 94; safety and long- term use of, 93-94; side effects of, 93; suppressive therapy, 88-90. *See also* treatments

TV commercials, 116
type-specific serologic tests
    (TSSTs), 54-57; Biokit test, 57;
    Captia test, 57; HerpeSelect
    tests, 55-57, 63; Western blot
    test, 54-55
Tzanck smear, 51

U

umbilication, 167
Updated Herpes Handbook, The,
    181
urinary-tract infections, 59
urinating into water, 98-99

V

vaccines, 99-100; for herpes
    simplex virus type 2, 100; for
    human papillomavirus, 164-
    165
vaginal delivery, 72
valacyclovir (Valtrex), 85, 86, 88,
    91, 187
varicella-zoster virus (VZV),
    13, 15-19; commonly asked
    questions about, 17-19; herpes
    simplex distinguished from,
    16-17
Varivax vaccine, 18
viral culture, 48-50
viral shedding, 19-20, 28, 41-42,
    158
viral STIs, 162-168; hepatitis
    B virus, 166-167; hepatitis

C virus, 165-166; human
    papillomavirus, 162-165;
    molluscum contagiosum, 167-
    168

W

Wald, Anna, 28, 38, 109
Web resources: diagnostic tests,
    186-187; medical information,
    180-183; networking sites,
    183-185; online dating, 185;
    patient medicine assistance,
    187-188; research studies, 187.
    See also Internet
WebMD website, 2, 183-184
Western blot test, 54-55
Westover Heights Clinic, 181
women's issues, 69-81; birth
    control, 79; breastfeeding,
    77; cervical cancer, 78-79;
    diagnosis of genital herpes,
    47; internal reproductive
    organs, 69-70; pregnancy
    and childbirth, 70-78, 80,
    81; questions and answers
    pertaining to, 79-81;
    susceptibility to genital herpes,
    27

Z

Zostavax vaccine, 16, 18, 19
Zovirax (acyclovir), 84-85, 86,
    88, 91, 95

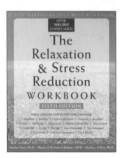
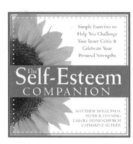
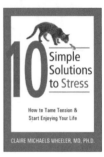
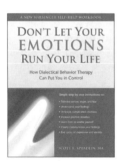
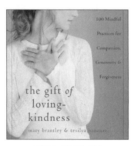
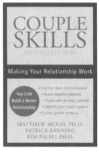